Textbook of Embryology, Anatomy, Physiology, Histology and Tooth Morphology

Textbook of Human Oral Embryology, Anatomy, Physiology, Histology and Tooth Morphology

KMK Masthan MDS
Professor and Head
Department of Oral Pathology and
Vice Principal (Academics)
Sree Balaji Dental College and Hospital, Chennai
Tamil Nadu, India

JAYPEE BROTHERS MEDICAL PUBLISHERS (P) LTD
Chennai • St Louis (USA) • Panama City (Panama) • London (UK) • New Delhi
Ahmedabad • Bengaluru • Hyderabad • Kochi • Kolkata • Lucknow • Mumbai • Nagpur

Published by
Jitendar P Vij
Jaypee Brothers Medical Publishers (P) Ltd

Corporate Office
4838/24 Ansari Road, Daryaganj, **New Delhi** - 110002, India,
Phone: +91-11-43574357, Fax: +91-11-43574314

Registered Office
B-3 EMCA House, 23/23B Ansari Road, Daryaganj, **New Delhi** - 110 002, India
Phones: +91-11-23272143, +91-11-23272703, +91-11-23282021
+91-11-23245672, Rel: +91-11-32558559, Fax: +91-11-23276490, +91-11-23245683
e-mail: jaypee@jaypeebrothers.com, Website: www.jaypeebrothers.com

Offices in India

- **Ahmedabad**, Phone: Rel: +91-79-32988717, e-mail: ahmedabad@jaypeebrothers.com
- **Bengaluru**, Phone: Rel: +91-80-32714073, e-mail: bangalore@jaypeebrothers.com
- **Chennai**, Phone: Rel: +91-44-32972089, e-mail: chennai@jaypeebrothers.com
- **Hyderabad**, Phone: Rel:+91-40-32940929, e-mail: hyderabad@jaypeebrothers.com
- **Kochi**, Phone: +91-484-2395740, e-mail: kochi@jaypeebrothers.com
- **Kolkata**, Phone: +91-33-22276415, e-mail: kolkata@jaypeebrothers.com
- **Lucknow**, Phone: +91-522-3040554, e-mail: lucknow@jaypeebrothers.com
- **Mumbai**, Phone: Rel: +91-22-32926896, e-mail: mumbai@jaypeebrothers.com
- **Nagpur**, Phone: Rel: +91-712-3245220, e-mail: nagpur@jaypeebrothers.com

Overseas Offices

- **North America Office, USA,** Ph: 001-636-6279734,
  e-mail: jaypee@jaypeebrothers.com, anjulav@jaypeebrothers.com
- **Central America Office, Panama City, Panama,** Ph: 001-507-317-0160,
  e-mail: cservice@jphmedical.com   Website: www.jphmedical.com
- **Europe Office, UK,** Ph: +44 (0) 2031708910, e-mail: dholman@jpmedical.biz

Textbook of Human Oral Embryology, Anatomy, Physiology, Histology and Tooth Morphology

© 2010, Jaypee Brothers Medical Publishers

All rights reserved. No part of this publication should be reproduced, stored in a retrieval system, or transmitted in any form or by any means: electronic, mechanical, photocopying, recording, or otherwise, without the prior written permission of the author and the publisher.

This book has been published in good faith that the material provided by author is original. Every effort is made to ensure accuracy of material, but the publisher, printer and author will not be held responsible for any inadvertent error (s). In case of any dispute, all legal matters are to be settled under Delhi jurisdiction only.

First Edition: **2010**

ISBN 978-81-8448-892-0

Typeset at JPBMP typesetting unit

Printed at Replika Press Pvt. Ltd.

To

My daughter Shafeeka

Prof C Bhasker Rao
MDS, FDSRCPS
Principal, SDM College of
Dental Sciences & Hospital
Vice President, Dental Council of India

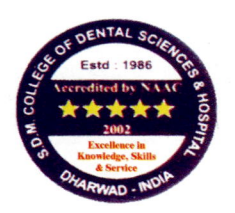

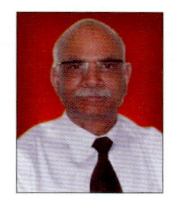

Foreword

I am pleased to introduce Dr KMK Masthan's *Textbook of Human Oral Embryology, Anatomy, Physiology, Histology and Tooth Morphology* to the student community. A concise presentation of this book will be of immense help to the students pursuing graduate studies. A few topics like role of calcium, effects of hormones on the oral structures, dental anatomy, ganglion and cranial nerves have been added to the textbook making it more informative. I am sure it will benefit all the students and the editor deserves a hearty congratulation for all the efforts that went in creating the *Textbook of Human Oral Embryology, Anatomy, Physiology, Histology and Tooth Morphology.*

Prof C Bhasker Rao

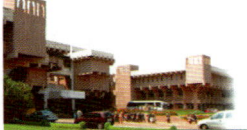

Preface

To understand oral diseases, the dental student needs to have a thorough knowledge of the anatomy, embryology, physiology and histology of oral structures. Therefore, in this book, I have made an attempt to present oral histology, oral embryology, tooth anatomy and oral physiology in a very simple and easy-to-understand manner. The purpose of this book is mainly to provide the undergraduate students an easy reference for covering a voluminous subject in lucid and simple language. I am especially grateful to Dr JP Rajguru, Dr Shankargouda Patil and Dr Shyam Sundar Behura my postgraduate students, Dr KT Shanmugam, MDS and Dr K Ramesh my faculty members for their spade work in compiling this book. Suggestions and feedback are welcome at *masthankmk@yahoo.com*

KMK Masthan
M Sathish Kumar
N Aravindha Babu

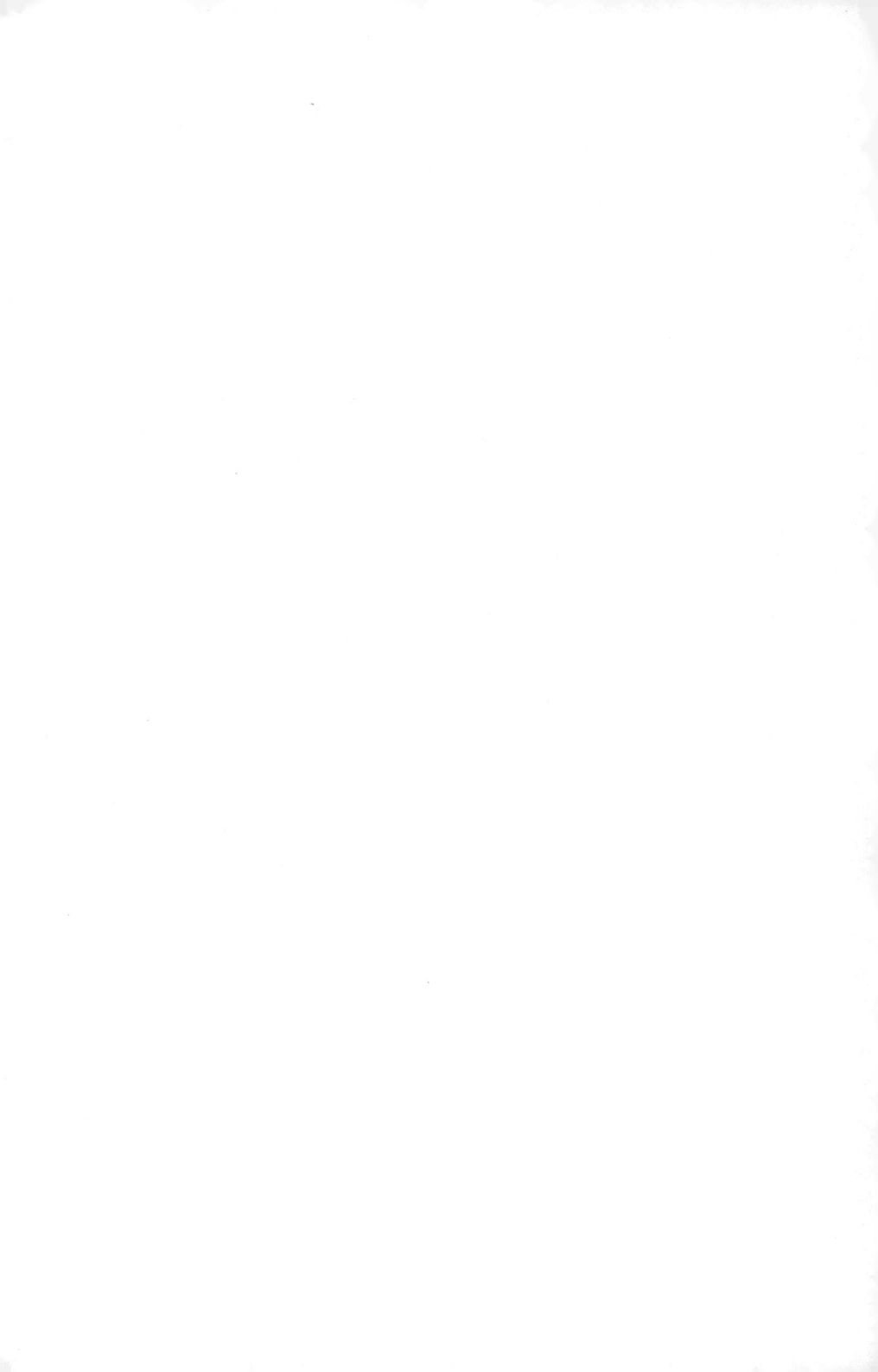

Contents

Section 1: Oral Embryology and Histology

1. Development of Face and Oral Cavity 3
2. Development and Growth of Teeth 17
3. Enamel 28
4. Dentin 42
5. Pulp 56
6. Cementum (Substantia Ossea) 70
7. Periodontal Ligament 76
8. Alveolar Process 83
9. Oral Mucous Membrane 90
10. Salivary Glands 105
11. Maxillary Sinus 120
12. Temporomandibular Joint 125
13. Tooth Eruption 132
14. Shedding of Deciduous Teeth 140

Section 2: Oral Physiology

15. Age Changes in Dental Tissues and Jaws 147
16. Effects of Hormones on the Oral Structures 153
17. Role of Calcium 177

Section 3: Dental Anatomy

18. Introduction of Dentition 185

Section 4: Histochemistry

19. Histochemistry of Oral Tissue 253
20. Microtechnique 261

Index 269

Section 1

Oral Embryology and Histology

Development of Face and Oral Cavity

Chapter 1

INTRODUCTION

The human somatic cell is diploid with 46 chromosomes (i.e. 23 pairs of chromosomes) of which 22 pairs are autosomes and one pair of sex chromosome (XX in female and XY in male). The germ cells or gametes are haploid cells (i.e. 23 chromosomes). During fertilization the male and female gamete unite to form the zygote (diploid).

The zygote formed undergoes mitosis repeatedly to form the embryo which later develops into an organism. Thus, all somatic cells in a multicellular organism are descendants of one original cell, the fertilized egg or zygote. Mitosis produces two daughter cells per cycle and their genetic content is identical to mother cell.

Gametogenesis (formation of gametes) occurs only in specialized cells (germ line) of the reproductive organs (gonads). In human, the testes are male gonads and the ovaries are female gonads. Gamete cells are produced through the process of mitosis. Mitosis consists of two specialized, consecutive cell divisions in which the chromosome number of resulting cells is reduced from a diploid (2n) to a haploid (n) number. The number of chromosomes must be reduced by half during gametogenesis in order to maintain the chromosome number and characteristic of the species after fertilization.

4 Oral Embryology and Histology

PRENATAL DEVELOPMENT

This occupies 10 lunar months.
- Early development has been divided into 23 stages on a combination of external features and the development of internal systems.

There is a measurement known as **(crown-rump length)** which is used to know the development of the embryo.

Prenatal development is divided into 3 stages
- First two stages when combined, constitute the embryonic stage of development and, 3rd stage is the fetal stage of development.
- First phase is 4 weeks of development. It involves the cellular proliferation and migration with some differentiation of cell population. Few congenital defect starts from this stage.
- Second phase is next 4 weeks and is largely characterized by the differentiation of cell (formation of external and internal structures), i.e. morphogenesis. This is vulnerable period of development for the embryo because it involves many intricate embryologic processes. During this period, many recognized congenital defect develop.

From the end of the second phase further development is largely a matter of growth and maturation and the embryo is now called a "FETUS".

After fertilization, a phase of rapid proliferation and migration of cells with little or no differentiation is seen. This stage lasts until 3 germ layers are formed.

Morula → Blastocyst → Trophoblast cells and embryoblast.

The embryoblast rapidly differentiates into 2 layers, so that at about 8 days an outer ectodermal and an inner endodermal layers can be distinguished.

FORMATION OF THE NEURAL TUBE

The nervous system develops as a thickening within the ectodermal layer at the head end of the embryo. This thickening

Development of Face and Oral Cavity

constitutes the neural plate, which rapidly forms raised margins that is neural folds.

Later a midline depression is formed called neural groove. The neural folds eventually fuse so that a neural tube separates from the ectoderm forming the floor of the amniotic cavity with mesoderm intervening.

Neural tube forms brain and spinal cord. A group of cells can be distinguished differentiating at the crest of the neural folds.

These cells separate from the fold and are known as neural crest cells.

In the mammalian embryo this same group of cells separate from the lateral aspect of the neural plate rather than its crest.

Functions

These cells have the capacity to differentiate extensively within developing embryo giving raise to number of structures like sensory ganglia, sympathetic neurons, Schwann cells, meninges and the cartilage of branchial arches.

It also forms most of the embryonic connective tissue in the facial region.

A proper migration of neural crest is essential for the development of the face and teeth.

Molecular biology and immunocytochemistry have helped to explain the processes of performing induction and competence.

Using probes composed of specific nucleic acid sequences, recombinant DNA technology can identify not only specific genes but also whether genes are exceptionally active.

By using specific antibodies for specific proteins, immunocytochemistry provides precise identification and localization of molecules with in a cell.

Examples of growth factors implicated in craniofacial development and tooth morphogenesis:

1. Transforming growth factor—Beta (TGF-β)
    i. TGF-β-1-5

6 Oral Embryology and Histology

    ii. Bone morphogenetic protein (BMP) (2-8)
    iii. Growth differentiation factor (GDF) (1-7).
2. Epidermal growth factor (EGF):
    i. EGF
    ii. TGF- α (Alpha)
    iii. Amphiregulin
    iv. Heparin - binding EGF
3. Fibroblast growth factor (FGF) (1-8)
4. Insulin-like growth factor (IGF) (1-2)
5. Platelet derived growth factor (PDGF) and B
6. Neurotrophins:
    i. Nerve growth factor (NGF)
    ii. Brain derived neurotrophic factor (BDNF)
    iii. Neurotrophins (NT) (3-4).

FORMATION OF THE THREE-LAYERED EMBRYO

At about day 8 of gestation, the cells of the embryoblast differentiate into a two-layered disk called bilaminar germ disk.

Cells situated dorsally or ectodermal layer are columnar and recognize to form the amniotic cavity.

On ventral aspect, the endodermal layer are cuboidal and form the roof of a second cavity, i.e. secondary yolk sac, which develops from the migration of peripheral cells of the extra-embryonic endodermal layer.

This configuration is completed after 2 weeks of development.

During this time the axis of the embryo is establised and is represented by a slight enlargement of the ectodermal and endodermal cells at the head end of the embryo in a region known as prochordal plate.

Firm union exist between the ectodermal and endodermal cells at the prochordal plate.

During the 3rd week of development the bilaminar embryonic disk is converted to a trilaminar disk.

The floor of the amniotic cavity is formed by ectoderm and within it a structure called primitive streak develops along the midline.

Development of Face and Oral Cavity   7

This is a narrow groove with slightly bulging area on each side.

The rostral end of the streak finishes in a small depression called the primitive node or pit.

Cells of the ectodermal layer divide at the node and migrate between the ectoderm and endoderm to form a solid column that pushes forward as far as the prochordal plate.

Through canalization of this cord of cells, the notochord is formed in the primitive embryo.

Along the side of the primitive streak, cells of the ectodermal layer divide and migrate toward the streak, they invaginate and spread laterally between the ectoderm and endoderm. This layer is called mesoderm.

Cells that accumulate inferior to the prochordal plate as a result of this migration gives rise to the cardiac plate.

FOLDING OF THE EMBRYO

The embryo folds in its two axis:
  (i) Rostrocaudal or cephalocaudal axis
  (ii) Lateral axis

The head fold is critical to the formation of a primitive stomatodeum or oral cavity, through this fold ectoderm comes to line the stomatodeum, with the stomatodeum separated from the gut by the buccopharyngeal membrane.

DERIVATIVES OF GERM LAYERS AND NEURAL CREST

A. Ectoderm	→ Neuroectoderm	→ Posterior pituitary gland, pineal body retina, central nervous system.
	Surface ectoderm →	Epidermis, hair, nail, cutaneous glands, mammary glands, anterior pituitary gland, parenchyma of salivary glands, enamel of teeth, lens, inner ear
B. Mesoderm	→ Paraxial	→ Muscles of trunk, skeleton (except skull), dermis of skin

Contd[a]

Contd^a

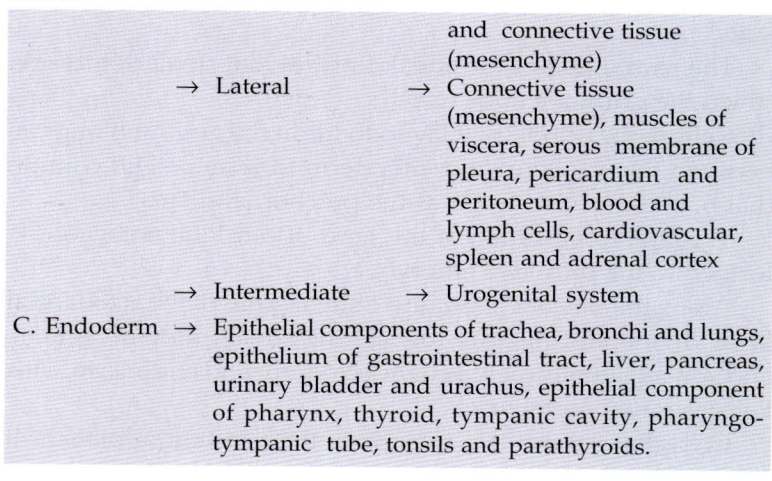

		and connective tissue (mesenchyme)
	→ Lateral	→ Connective tissue (mesenchyme), muscles of viscera, serous membrane of pleura, pericardium and peritoneum, blood and lymph cells, cardiovascular, spleen and adrenal cortex
	→ Intermediate	→ Urogenital system
C. Endoderm	→	Epithelial components of trachea, bronchi and lungs, epithelium of gastrointestinal tract, liver, pancreas, urinary bladder and urachus, epithelial component of pharynx, thyroid, tympanic cavity, pharyngotympanic tube, tonsils and parathyroids.

HEAD FORMATION

The neural tube is produced by the formation and fusion of the neural folds, which sink beneath the surface ectoderm.

Anterior portion of this neural tube expands greatly as the forebrain, mid brain, and hind brain form. But a small amount of mesenchyme always remains between the developing brain and the surface epithelium except where the olfactory, orbital and otic placodes form.

The part of the hindbrain develops a series of eight bulges, i.e. the rhombomeres.

Lateral to the neural tube is paraxial mesoderm, which partially segments postnatally to form seven somotomeres and fully segments caudally to form somites, the first in the series being the occipital somites.

Migration of neural crest cells provides the embryonic connective tissue needed for craniofacial development.

These neural crest cells arise from the midbrain and the first two rhombomeres as 2 streams.

The first stream migrates forward and intermingles and reinforces the mesenchyme situated beneath the expanding forebrain.

This stream provides nuclei of the connective tissue associated with the face.

The second stream is directed to the first arch and is derived from the neuroectoderm of the midbrain and the first two rhombomeres.

BRANCHIAL ARCHES AND THE PRIMITIVE MOUTH

When stomatodeum first forms it is delimited rostrally by the frontal prominence and caudally by developing cardiac bulge.

Buccopharyngeal membrane separates the stomatodeum from the foregut, but this soon breaks directly with foregut.

Laterally the stomatodeum communicates directly with the foregut.

Laterally the stomatodeum becomes limited by the first pair of pharyngeal or branchial arches.

Six cylindrical thickenings thus form and expands from the lateral wall of the pharynx passes beneath the floor of the pharynx and approach their anatomic counter parts expanding from the opposite side.

The arches progressively separate the primitive stomatodeum from the developing heart.

Arches are seen clearly as bulges on the lateral aspect of the embryo and are separated externally by small clefts called branchial grooves.

On the inner aspect pharyngeal pouches are seen.

FATE OF GROOVES AND POUCHES

All these grooves and pouches gives some basic structures, i.e. the derivatives of the organs.

First, second and third branchial arches play an important role in the development of the face, mouth and tongue.

Primitive stomatodeum is at first bounded above (rostrally) by frontal prominence, below (caudally) by the developing heart and laterally by the first branchial arches.

With spread of the arches midventrally the cardiac plate is eliminated from the stomatodeum covering the mesenchyme of the first, second and third branchial arches.

At about 24 days the first branchial arch estabilizes.

The stomatodeum is limited cranially by the frontal prominence covering the rapidly expanding forebrain, laterally by the newly formed maxillary process and ventrally by first arch called mandibular process.

DEVELOPMENT OF THE FACE

Early development is seen by the proliferation and migration of ectomesenchyme involved in the formation of the primitive nasal cavities.

At 28 days localized thickenings develop within the ectoderm of the frontal prominence, just rostral to the opening of the stomatodeum called olfactory placode.

Rapid proliferation of the underlying mesenchyme around the placodes bulge the frontal eminence forward and also produces a horse-shoe shaped bridge that converts the olfactory placode into the nasal pit.

The lateral arm of the horse-shoe is called the lateral nasal process and the medial arm is the medial nasal process.

Frontal and nasal prominence join and form frontonasal process.

The medial nasal processes of both sides, together with the frontonasal process give rise to the middle portion of the nose, middle portion of the upper lip, and portion of the maxilla and primary palate.

The maxillary process pushes the medial nasal process toward the midline.

In this way the upper lip is formed from the maxillary process and the lateral face of the medial nasal process.

Lower lip is formed by merging of the two stream of ectomesenchyme of the mandibular process.

The merging of the two medial nasal process results in the formation of the part of the maxilla carrying the incisor teeth and the primary palate as well as part of lip.

An usual type of fusion occurs between the maxillary process and the lateral nasal process as with most other processes

Development of Face and Oral Cavity

associated with facial development, the maxillary and lateral nasal process, initially are separated by a deep furrow.

The epithelium in the floor of the groove between them forms a solid core that separates from the surface and eventually canalizes to form a nasolacrimal duct. Once the duct has separated the two processes merge by infilling of the mesenchyme.

Face develops between the 24-28th days of gestation. By this time some of the epithelium covering the facial processes already can be distinguished as odontogenic or tooth forming.

On the inferior border of the maxillary process and superior border of mandibular arch, the epithelium begins to proliferate and thicken called odontogenic epithelium.

Then the primary epithelial band is observed. It is an arch shaped continuous plate of odontogenic epithelium that forms in the upper jaw from 4 zones of epithelial proliferation, the middle two associated with medial nasal process.

Two other zone one in each mandibular process form the primary epithelial band of lower jaw.

DEVELOPMENT OF SECONDARY PALATE

Only after development of the secondary palate the oral and nasal cavity is distinct.

It develops from primary and secondary components.

Formation of secondary palate starts at 7-8 weeks and completes around the 3rd month of gestation.

Three out growth appears in the oral cavity:
(i) Nasal septum
(ii) Two palatine shelves

Nasal septum grows downward from the frontonasal process along the midline and palatine shelves one from each side extend from the maxillary processes towards the midline.

The shelves are directed first downward on each side of the tongue. After the 7th week of development, the tongue is withdrawn from between the shelves, which now elevate and fuse with each other above the tongue and with the primary palate.

Two palatal shelves converge and fuse along the midline, thus separating primitive cavity into nasal and oral cavities.

Closure of the secondary palate involves an intrinsic force in the palatine shelves the nature of which has not been determined yet.

Between 7-8 weeks the tongue and mandible are small and is positioned behind the lower lip.

By 9th week the upper facial complex has lifted away from the thorax and thus permits the tongue and lower jaw to grow forward, so that it is balanced.

As two palatine shelves meet, adhesion of the epithelia occurs. So that the epithelium of one shelf becomes indistinguishable from that of the other and a midline epithelial seam forms.

To achieve this fusion, DNA synthesis ceases within the epithelium some 24-36 hours before epithelial contact.

These cells have a carbohydrate - rich surface coat that permits ready adhesion and the formation of junctions to achieve fusion of the processes.

DEVELOPMENT OF THE TONGUE

It develops at about 4 weeks.

The pharyngeal arches meet in the midline beneath the primitive mouth.

Local proliferation of the mesenchyme gives rise to a number of swellings in the floor of the mouth.

Tuberculum impar arises in the midline in mandibular process and flanked by two other bulges, the lingual swellings.

Lateral lingual swellings quickly enlarge and merge with each other and the tuberculum impar to form a large mass from which the mucous membrane of the anterior 2/3rd of the tongue is formed.

Root of the tongue arises from the hypobranchial eminence, a large midline swelling developed from the mesenchyme of the 3rd arch.

Development of Face and Oral Cavity

The mesenchyme of 3rd arch rapidly over grows the second arch, which thereby is excluded from further involvement in the development of the tongue.

Hypobranchial eminence gives rise to posterior 1/3rd of the tongue.

It has been stated by some authors that hypobranchial eminence has 2 parts.

(i) Anterior copula → which gives origin to the mucosa covering the root of the tongue.

(ii) A hypobranchial eminence → which gives rise to the epiglottis

The tongue separates from the floor of the mouth by downgrowth of the ectoderm, which subsequently degenerates to form the lingual sulcus and gives the tongue mobility.

Muscles of the tongue arise from occipital somites, which is supplied by 12th cranial nerve.

Because the mucosa of the anterior 2/3rd of the tongue is derived from the 1st arch, it is supplied by 5th cranial nerve whereas the mucosa of the posterior 1/3rd derived from 3rd arch and it is supplied by 9th cranial nerve.

DEVELOPMENT OF THE SKULL

Skull consists of cranial vault, cranial base and face.

Development is seen in approximately 12- week old human fetus.

The cartilagenous skull is represented by nasal and orbital cartilages and the petrosal and occipital bones from the original neurocranium.

The petrosal bone has incorporated the otic capsule. The only part of the viscerocranium contributing to the skull are the terminal parts of first and second arch cartilages, which become ear ossicles.

Thus, cartilagenous bone undergoes endochondral ossification

Membranous bone formed directly in mesenchyme with no cartilagenous precursor, forms the cranial vault and face.

14   Oral Embryology and Histology

DEVELOPMENT OF MANDIBLE

Derived from first branchial arch.

Meckel's cartilage develops the lower jaw.

It has close positional relationship to the developing mandible but makes no contribution to it.

At 6th week of development this cartilage extends as a hyaline cartilagenous rod, surrounded by a fibrocapsule, from the developing ear region to the midline of the fused mandibular processes.

Two cartilages meet at the midline but are separated by a thin band of mesenchyme. Mandibular branch of 5th cranial nerve has a close relation to Meckel's cartilage beginning 2/3rd of the way along the length of the cartilage.

At this part the mandibular nerve divides into lingual and inferior alveolar branches, which tour along the medial and lateral aspects of the cartilage.

Inferior alveolar nerve further divides into incisor and mental branch.

On the lateral aspect of Meckel's cartilage, during 6th week of embryonic development, a condensation of mesenchyme occurs in the angle formed by the division of inferior alveolar and its incisor and mental branches.

At 7th week, intramembranous ossification begins in this condensation forming the first bone of mandible.

From the center of ossification bone formation spreads anteriorly and posteriorly.

This spread of new bone formation occurs anteriorly along the lateral aspect of Meckel's cartilage forming a trough that consists of lateral and medial plates that unit beneath the incisor nerve.

The two separate centers of ossification remain separated at the mandibular symphysis until shortly after birth.

The trough is soon converted into a canal as bone forms over the nerve joining the lateral and medial plates.

Backward ossification on lateral aspect of Meckel's cartilage forms canal that contains the inferior alveolar nerve.

Ramus of the mandible develops by a rapid spread of ossification posteriorly into the mesenchyme of first arch running away from Meckel's cartilage.

This point of divergence forms lingula in adult mandible, the point at which inferior alveolar nerve enters the body of mandible.

Thus by 10th week, the rudimentary mandible formed almost entirely by membranous ossification with little direct involvement of Meckel's cartilage.

Further growth of the mandible until birth is influenced by appearance of 3 secondary cartilages and the development of muscular attachments:
 (i) The condylar cartilage
 (ii) The coronoid cartilage
 (iii) The symphyseal cartilage.

DEVELOPMENT OF MAXILLA

It develops from a center of ossification in the mesenchyme of the maxillary process of the first arch.

Center of ossification is associated closely with the cartilage of the nasal capsule.

From this center, bone formation spreads posteriorly below the orbit toward the developing zygoma and anteriorly towards the incisor region.

Ossification also spreads superiorly to form the frontal process.

There will be formation of trough for infraorbital nerve from this a downward extension of bone forms the lateral plate for the maxillary tooth germs.

A secondary cartilage also contribute to the development of the maxilla.

Body of the maxilla is relatively small because the maxillary sinus has not developed.

This sinus forms during the 16th week.

16 Oral Embryology and Histology

Common Features of Jaw Development

Both begin from a single layer of membranous ossification related to a nerve and to a primary cartilage.
- Both form a neural element related to the developing teeth.
- Both develop secondary cartilages to assist in their growth.

DEVELOPMENT OF TEMPOROMANDIBULAR JOINT

TMJ is an articulation between two bones initially formed from membranous centers of ossification.

Before the condylar cartilage forms, a broad band of undifferentiated mesenchyme exists between the developing ramus of mandible and developing squamous tympanic bone.

With formation of the condylar cartilage, this band is reduced rapidly in width and converted into a dense strip of mesenchyme.

The mesenchyme immediately adjacent to this strip breaks down to form the joint cavity and the strip becomes the articular disk.

After 8th week, development is essentially a matter of growth.

Development and Growth of Teeth

Chapter 2

DENTAL LAMINA

Two-three weeks after the rupture of buccopharyngeal membrane, when the embryo is 6 weeks old, certain areas of basal cells of oral ectoderm proliferate at rapid rate than cells of adjacent areas, thus forming the dental lamina, which is a band of epithelium that has invaded the underlying ectomesenchyme along each of the horse-shoe shaped future dental arches.

Development of the 1st permanent molar is initiated at 4th month in utero.

Development of second molar is initiated at first year after birth.

The distal proliferation of the dental lamina is responsible for the location of the germs of the permanent molars in the ramus of the mandible and the tuberosity of the maxilla.

The successors of the deciduous teeth develop from a lingual extension

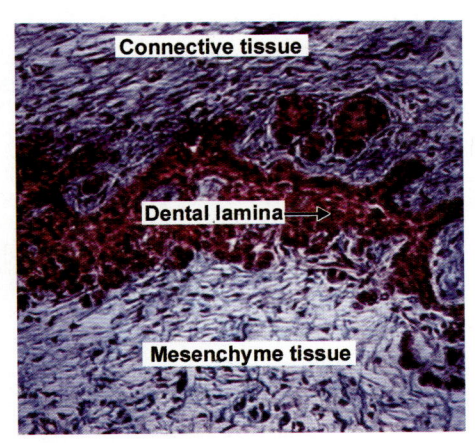

Fig. 2.1: Development of dental lamina

of the free end of the dental lamina opposite to the enamel organ of each deciduous tooth.

The lingual extension of the dental lamina is named the successional lamina and develops from the fifth month *in utero* (permanent central incisor) to the tenth month of age (second premolar).

Fate of Dental Lamina

The total activity of dental lamina extends over a period of 5 years.

The dental lamina may still be active in the 3rd molar region after it has disappeared elsewhere. As the teeth continue to develop, they lose their connection with the dental lamina.

Remnants of the dental lamina (cell rests of serrae) persist as epithelial pearls or islands within the jaw as well as in the gingiva.

TOOTH DEVELOPMENT

At certain points of the dental lamina, ectodermal cells multiply more rapidly and form little knobs that grow into the underlying mesenchyme. These represents areas of 10 mandibular and 10 maxillary deciduous teeth in their respective arches.

Each of these little knobs represent beginning of enamel organ.

First to appear are the anterior mandibular incisors.

Developmental Stages

Several 'morphologic' stages named after the shape of the epithelial part of the tooth germ.
a. Bud stage
b. Cap stage
c. Bell stages
  – Early
  – Advanced

Bud Stage

Epithelium of dental lamina is separated from the underlying ectomesenchyme by a basement membrane.

With differentiation of each dental lamina, round swelling arises at 10 different points in each jaw.

These represent the future position of deciduous teeth and are primordia of enamel organs, the tooth buds.

Thus, development of the tooth germs are initiated and cells continue to proliferate faster than adjacent cells.

Main function of certain epithelial cells of tooth bud is to form enamel - hence *enamel organ*.

In bud stage, enamel organ consists of:
- Peripherally located low columnar cells.
- Centrally located polygonal cells.

Many cells of tooth bud and surrounding mesenchyme, undergo mitosis; due to this and migration of neural crest cells into the area, ectomesenchymal cells sorrounding the tooth bud condense.

This ectomesenchymal condensation subadjacent to the enamel organ is the *dental papilla*.

Condensed ectomesenchyme surrounding the tooth bud and dental papilla is called *dental sac*.

Dental papilla → Gives rise to dentin and the tooth pulp.

Dental sac → Gives rise to cementum, periodontal ligament and alveolar bone.

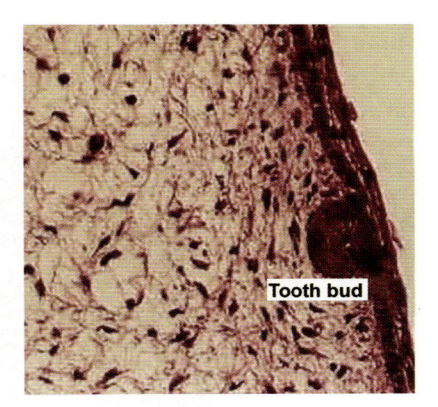

Fig. 2.2: Illustrates the earliest extension of the epithelium, called a tooth bud. The epithelia will continue to proliferate and form a process, shown in the following photograph

Cap Stage

As tooth bud proliferates, unequal growth in different

20 Oral Embryology and Histology

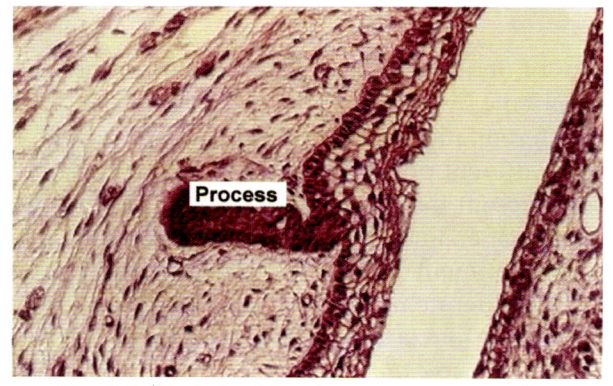

Fig. 2.3: Tooth bud forming process, extending in from dental lamina

parts of the tooth bud leads to a shallow invagination in the deeper surface of the bud leading to cap stage.

Peripheral cells of the cap are cuboidal, cover the convexity of the cap forming outer enamel epithelium.

Cells covering concavity are tall-columnar and they represent inner enamel epithelium

Outer enamel epithelium is separated from dental sac and inner enamel epithelium from dental papilla by a delicate basement membrane. Hemidesmosomes anchor the cells to basal lamina.

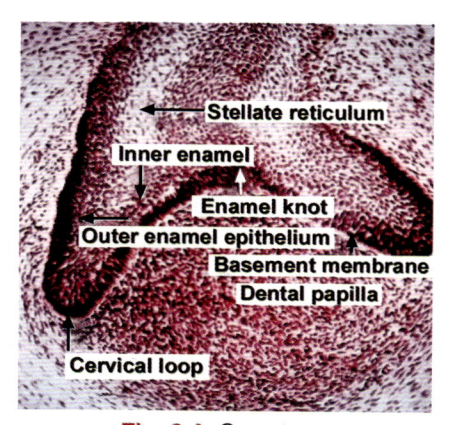

Fig. 2.4: Cap stage

Stellate Reticulum (Enamel Pulp)

Polygonal cells in center of epithelial enamel organ between outer and inner epithelium begin to separate as more intercellular fluid is produced and form a cellular network called the stellate reticulum.

The spaces between the cells are filled with a mucoid fluid rich in albumin, which gives a cushioning consistency that may support and protect delicate enamel- forming cells. Cells assume a branched reticular network.

Cells in the center of enamel organ are densely packed and form the enamel knot.

There arises a vertical extension from the enamel knot called enamel cord.

Both the structures are temporary and disappear before enamel formation.

Function of Enamel Knot and Cord

Act as a reservoir of dividing cells for the growing enamel organ.

Dental Papilla

Proliferating epithelium of enamel organ influences the ectomesenchymal enclosure by invaginated portion of inner enamel epithelium.

It condenses to form dental papilla which is the formative organ for dentin and primordium of dental pulp.

Dental papilla shows active budding of capillaries and mitotic figures and peripheral cells adjacent to inner enamel epithelium enlarge and differentiate into odontoblasts later.

Dental Sac

Marginal condensation of mesenchyme surrounding the enamel organ and dental papilla is dental sac which is dense and fibrous in the primitive stage and forms periodontal ligament, cementum and alveolar bone.

Bell Stage

As invagination of the epithelium deepens and its margins continue to grow, it assumes a 'Bell' shape.

In this stage, four types of epithelial cells can be distinguished by light microscope.
a. Inner enamel epithelium
b. Stratum intermedium
c. Stellate reticulum
d. Outer enamel epithelium

Inner Enamel Epithelium

Consists of a single layer of cells that differentiate into tall columnar cells prior to amelogenesis called ameloblasts, which are 4-5 µm width and 40 µm tall.

The cells are attached laterally by junctional complexes and to cells of stratum intermedium by desmosomes.

Cells of inner enamel epithelium exert an organizing influence on underlying mesenchymal cells in the dental papilla which later differentiate into odontoblasts.

Stratum Intermedium

Few layers of squamous cells form stratum intermedium between inner enamel epithelium and stellate reticulum.

Cells are closely attached by desmosomes and junctional complexes.
- High degree of metabolic activity is seen.
- This layer seems to be essential for enamel formation.

Stellate Reticulum

Expands by increase in intercellular fluid.

Cells are star-shaped, with long processes that anastamose with those of adjacent cells.

Before enamel formation, stellate reticulum collapses, reducing the distance between centrally situated ameloblasts and nutrient capillaries near outer enamel epithelium.

Outer Enamel Epithelium

Cells are flattened to low - cuboidal.

During and prior of enamel formation, smooth surface of outer enamel epithelium is laid in folds.

Between folds, the adjacent mesenchyme of the dental sac forms papilla that contains capillary loops thus providing nutritional supply to avascular enamel organ.

Dental Papilla

Before inner enamel epithelium forms enamel, the peripheral cells of the dental papilla differentiate to odontoblasts. They assume cuboid form initially later becomes tall columnar.

The basement membrane between enamel organ and dental papilla just prior to dentin formation is called membrana preformativa.

Dental Sac

With development of root, fibers of dental sac differentiate into periodontal fibers that become embedded in developing cementum and alveolar bone.

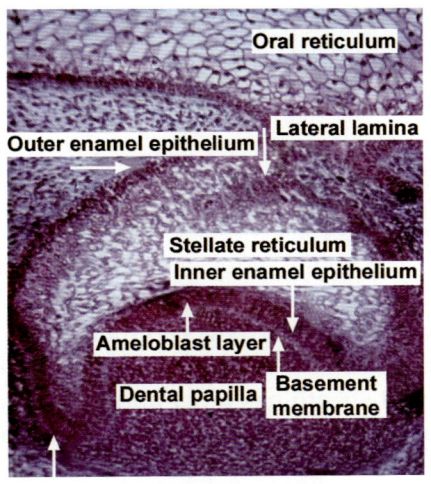

Fig. 2.5: Early bell stage

Advanced Bell Stage

The boundary between inner enamel epithelium and odontoblasts outlines the future dentino-enamel junction.

Cervical portion of enamel organ gives rise to Hertwig's epithelial root sheath.

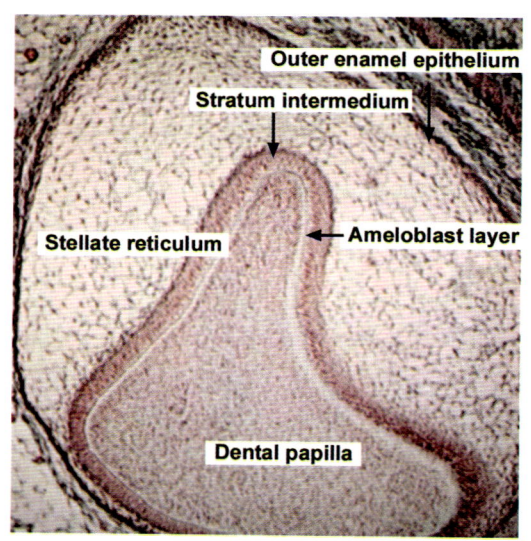

Fig. 2.6: Advance bell stage

HERTWIG'S EPITHELIAL ROOT SHEATH AND ROOT FORMATION

Root development begins after enamel and dentin formation has reached future cemento-enamel junction.

Enamel organ forms Hertwig's epithelial root sheath, which molds shape of roots and initiates radicular dentin formation

Hertwig's root sheath has inner and outer enamel epithelia without stratum intermedium and stellate reticulum.

The cells of inner enamel epithelia remains short, normal and don't produce enamel.

Development and Growth of Teeth 25

When these cells have induced differentiation of radicular cells into odontoblast, first layer of dentin has been laid down.

Hertwig's root sheath loses its structural continuity and its close relation to the surface of root.

The remnants of it persists near the external surface of the teeth in the periodontal ligament of erupted teeth called cell rests of Malassez.

Pronounced difference is seen in development of roots of one (or) multirooted teeth.

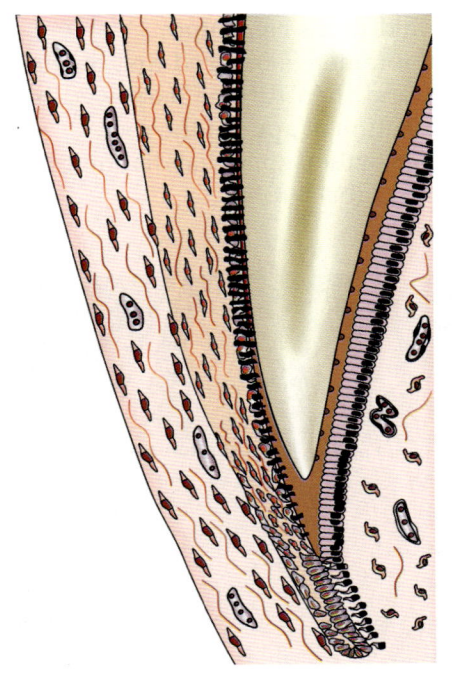

Fig. 2.7: Hertwig's epithelial root sheath

Before beginning of root formation, root sheath forms the epithelial diaphragm.

Outer and inner enamel epithelia bend at future cementoenamel junction in a horizontal plane.

26 Oral Embryology and Histology

Proliferation of cells of epithelial diaphragm is accompanied by proliferation of the cells of connective tissue of the pulp, which occurs adjacent to diaphragm.

Free end of diaphragm doesn't proliferate into connective tissue but proliferates coronally to epithelial diaphragm.

Differentiation of odontoblasts and formation of dentin, follows root sheath lengthening.

Connective tissue of dental sac surrounding the root sheath divides into double continuous epithelial layer.

Epithelium moves away from root surface of dentin. Connective tissue cells contact the surface and differentiate to cementoblasts and forms cementum.

Wide apical foramen is reduced first to width of diaphragmatic opening and then further narrowed by deposition of dentin and cementum at apex of the root.

Differential growth of epithelial diaphragm causes division of root trunk into 2 (or) 3 roots.

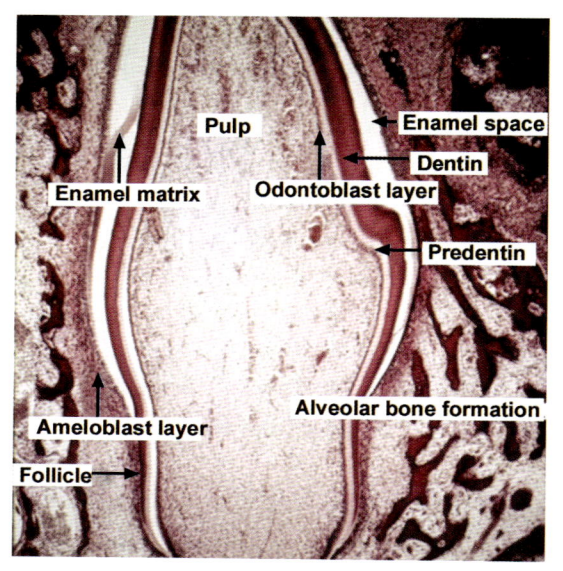

Fig. 2.8: Single rooted tooth formation

Development and Growth of Teeth 27

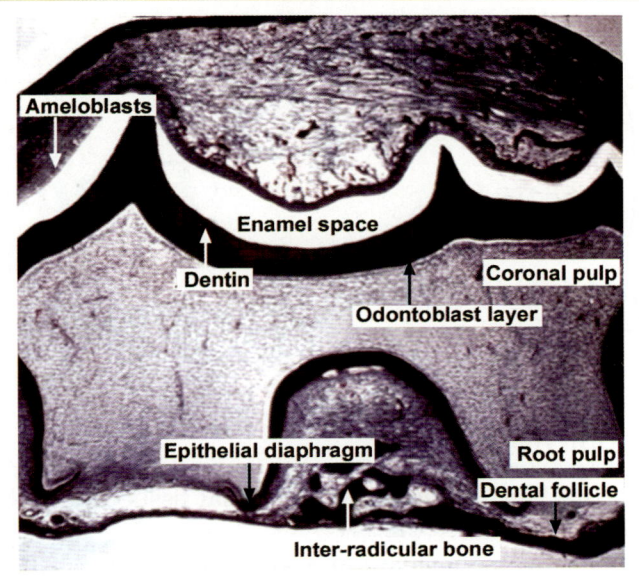

Fig. 2.9: Multirooted tooth formation

Long tongue-like extensions of horizontal diaphragm develop.

Two such extensions are seen in germs of lower molars and three are in upper molars.

Enamel

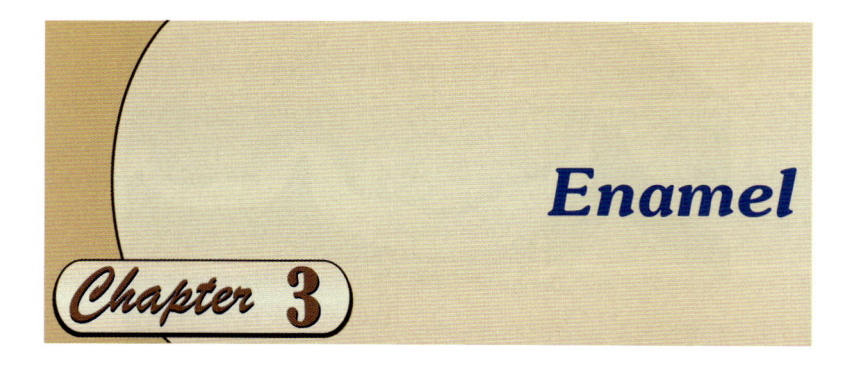

Chapter 3

INTRODUCTION

Enamel is a hard mineralized epithelial tissue of ectodermal origin.
- Enamel covers the anatomic crown of the tooth.
- Enamel is the only tissue that is totally acellular.

PHYSICAL PROPERTIES

Color

It appears bluish white or grayish at the thick opaque areas and yellowish white at the thin areas reflecting underlying dentin.

Hardness

It is the hardest structure of the body. Hardness varies from 5 to 8 Khn.

Hardness varies in different teeth and in different areas of the same tooth.

This variation depends on the degree of calcification, prism orientation, distribution of metallic ions.

Permeability

Enamel is selectively permeable.

The route of passage occurs mainly via the rod sheath, enamel lamellae, enamel tufts which are rich in organic content.

Density

Density decreases from the surface of the enamel to the dentino-enamel junction.
- It varies from 3.0 to 2.84 gm/ml.
- Permanent teeth have more density than deciduous teeth.

Thickness

Thickness varies over different parts of a tooth and from one type of tooth to another.

It is thickest over the cusps of the molars where it measures 2.5 mm and over incisal edges of incisors where it is 2.0 mm.

Tensile Strength and Compressibility

Elastic modulus is 19×10^6 psi, which indicates, it is brittle. It has low tensile strength of 11,000 psi which indicates its rigid structure.

Solubility

Enamel dissolves in acid media.

Solubility rate is influenced by certain ions and molecules such as fluorides, silver nitrate, zinc chloride, carbonates, organic matrix, etc.

CHEMICAL PROPERTIES

Enamel is composed of both Inorganic and Organic substances.

Mature enamel is made of 96% Inorganic and 4% Organic material and water.

Inorganic content is basically hydroxyapatite crystals and ions such as magnesium, lead and fluoride.

Organic material is mostly tyrosine-rich amelogenin, pectin and nonamelogenin proteins.

STRUCTURE OF ENAMEL

Enamel is composed of the following:
1. Enamel rods (Prisms)
2. Rod sheaths
3. Cementing inter-rod substance.

The basic structural unit of enamel is the enamel rod (prism).

The enamel rod is a very long, thin structure extending from the dentino-enamel junction to the surface of the enamel.

Enamel rods follow a tortuous course.

Each enamel rod appears to be encased in a rod sheath and the sheathed rods are cemented together by an inter rod substance.

Enamel rod is the most highly mineralized and the rod sheath the least mineralized.

Enamel rods have an average diameter of 4.5 mm.

Diameter of the rod increases from the dentino-enamel junction towards the enamel surface.

Number of enamel rods vary from 7.5 million in the mandibular incisors to 2.5 million in the maxillary molars.

In the cross-section enamel rods may apppear round or oval or hexagonal in shape.

Most often they have a keyhole configuration.

Each rod has a head and a tail. The 'head' is formed by one ameloblast and 'tail' is formed by 3 ameloblasts.

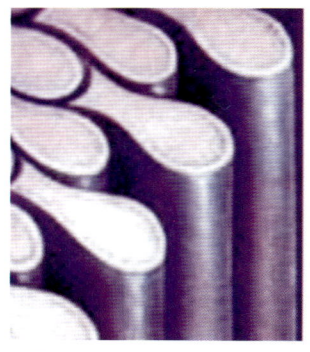

Fig. 3.1A: Keyhole pattern   **Fig. 3.1B:** Fish scale pattern

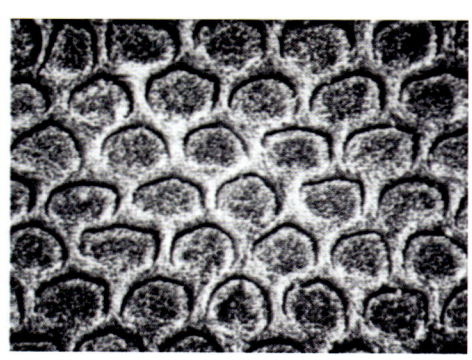

Enamel rods are arranged perpendicular to the DEJ, except in the cervical region where they are inclined towards gingiva.

The boundary where the crystals of the rod meet those of the inter rod substance is known as rod sheath.

Enamel crystals are 30 mm thick by 65 mm wide and several micrometers in length.

STRUCTURAL FEATURES OF ENAMEL

Incremental Lines of Retzius

In longitudinal sections of the teeth, these lines are seen as brownish bands that surround the tip of dentin.

In cross-section they appear as concentric rings.

Lines of Retzius represent incremental nature of enamel deposition.

These lines represent hypomineralized enamel.

An accentuated stria represents the disturbances at birth, is the neonatal line.

Neonatal lines can be seen in primary dentition and the first molar of the permanent dentition.

This line demarcates the prenatal and postnatal enamel.

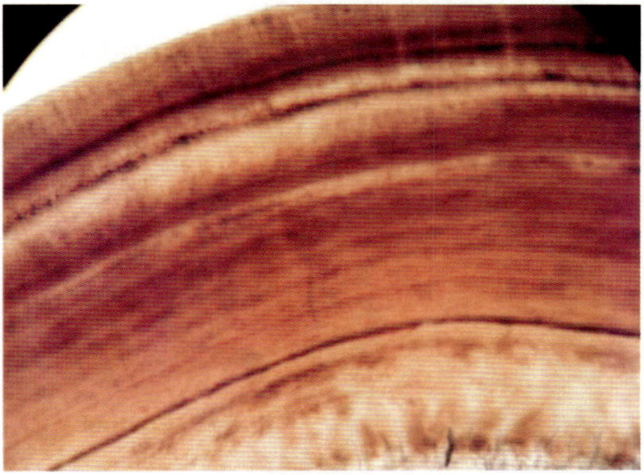

Fig. 3.2A: Incremental lines of Retzius in transverse section

32 Oral Embryology and Histology

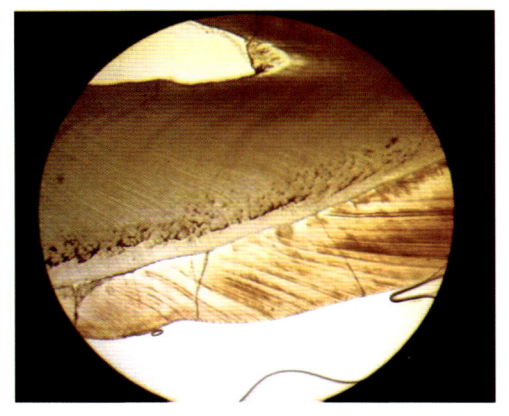

Fig. 3.2B: Incremental lines of Retzius in longitudinal section

Hunter-Schreger Bands

They are alternating dark and light zones seen in longitudinal ground sections when viewed under reflected light.

These bands originate at the dentino-enamel junction and pass outward traversing more than half of enamel.

These bands occur due to changes in rod direction.

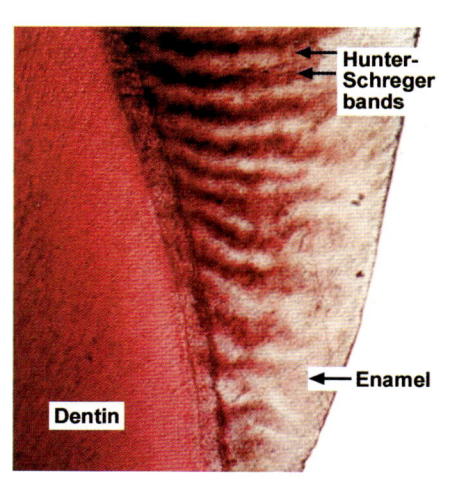

Fig. 3.3: Hunter-Schreger bands

Gnarled Enamel

Enamel rods below the cuspal and incisal region appear irregular, twisted and intertwisted, such a kind of enamel is called gnarled enamel.

Gnarled enamel extends throughout the thickness of enamel at the cusp tips and incisal edges.

Enamel Lamellae

They extend from the enamel surface towards the dentino - enamel junction.

They are hypomineralized structures.

They are seen in areas of tension where a short segment of the rod is not fully calcified.

They are classified into 3 types:

Type A

They are lamellae composed of poorly calcified rod segments.

Type B

They are lamellae consisting of degenerated cells.

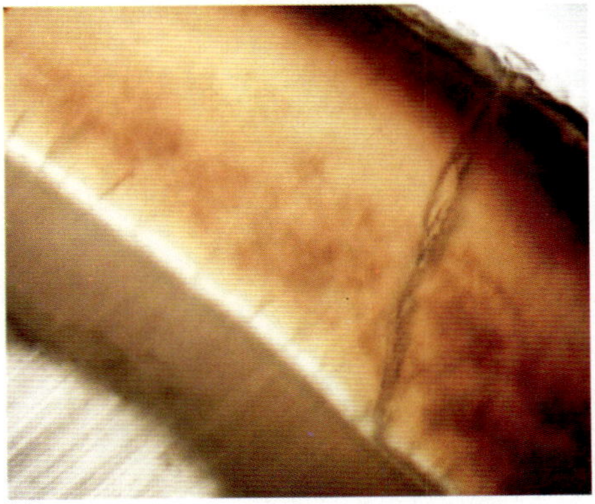

Fig. 3.4: Enamel lamellae

Type C

They are cracks seen in erupted teeth that are filled with organic matter or debris from saliva and is usually not cellular.

Enamel lamellae may be a site of weakness, which may form the pathway for bacterial invasion.

Enamel Tufts

They are organic structures that orginate at the dentino-enamel junction and extend into enamel for about one-third to one-fifth of its thickness.

Resemble tufts of grass and are areas where young enamel proteins are not completely transformed during maturation.

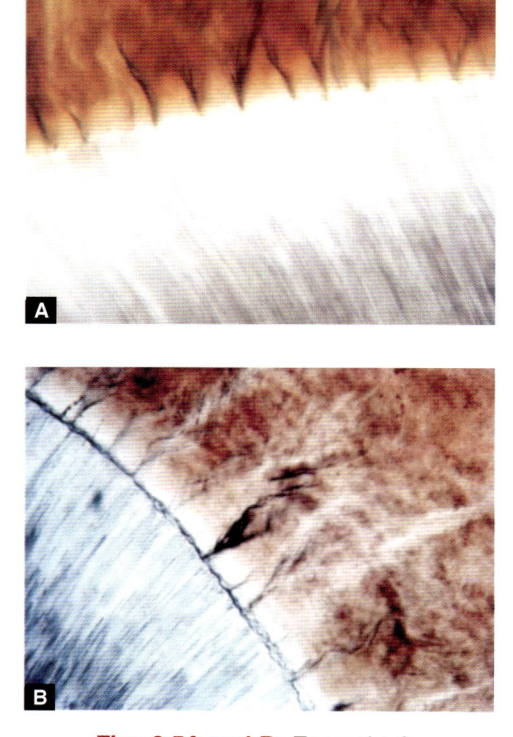

Figs 3.5A and B: Enamel tufts

Developmentally, they are formed due to the abrupt changes in the rod direction which lead to different ratio of inter rod and rod enamel, creating less mineralized and weakend planes.

Enamel Spindles

They are odontoblastic processes which cross the dentino-enamel junction and got entrapped in the enamel matrix.

Enamel spindles have an organic content higher than surrounding enamel.

They are randomly distributed along the dentino-enamel junction.

Often club shaped in ground sections.

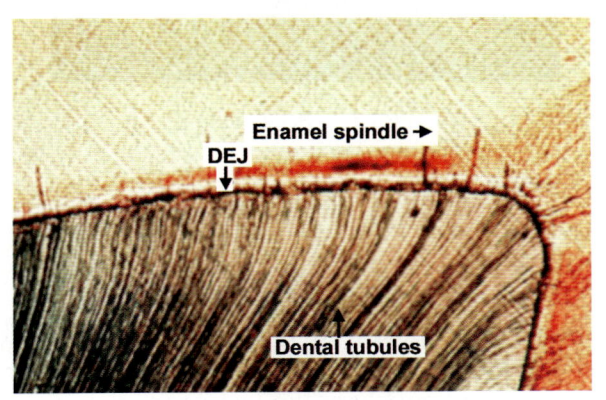

Fig. 3.6: Enamel spindles

SURFACE STRUCTURES

Perikymata

They are external manifestations of the striae of Retzius where they end in shallow furrows.

Seen prominently on the facial surface of the teeth, mostly in the middle and cervical thirds of the crown.

Are usually parallel to each other and to the cemento-enamel junction.

They are more numerous at the cervical area where they are about 30 per mm.

In the occlusal or incisal region they are 10 per mm.

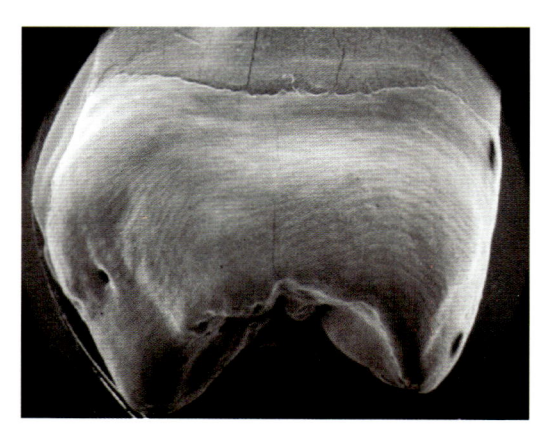

Fig. 3.7: Perikymata

Enamel Cuticle

The enamel cuticle or Nasmyth's membrane or primary cuticle is a structureless membrane seen on the crown of tooth, adhering firmly to its surface.

Seen in newly erupted teeth and is lost due to mastication. It is about 0.5 to 1.5 mm thick.

Primary enamel cuticle is the last product of the enamel forming ameloblasts and it becomes mineralized.

Secondary enamel cuticle covers the primary cuticle and is a product of the reduced enamel epithelium and is not mineralized.

The salivary pellicle seen over the enamel is a precipitate of salivary proteins.

LIFE CYCLE OF AMELOBLAST

Life span of the cells of the inner enamel epithelium can be divided into 6 stages:

Enamel 37

1. Morphogenic stage.
2. Organizing stage.
3. Formative stage.
4. Maturative stage.
5. Protective stage.
6. Desmolytic stage.

MORPHOGENIC STAGE

Before the Ameloblasts are fully differentiated and produce enamel, they interact with the adjacent mesenchymal cells, determining the shape of dentino-enamel junction and the crown.

The cells are short and columnar, with large oval nuclei that almost fill the cell body.

Golgi apparatus and the centrioles are located in the proximal end of the cell whereas the mitochondria are evenly dispersed throughtout the cytoplasm.

Terminal bars appear concomitantly with the migration of the mitochondria to the basal region of the cell.

The inner enamel epithelium is separated from the connective tissue of the dental papilla by a delicate basal lamina.

ORGANIZING STAGE

The inner enamel epithelium interacts with the adjacent connective tissue cells, which differentiate into odontoblasts.

The inner enamel epithelial cells become longer.

Reverse functional polarity of cells takes place by the migration of the centrioles and Golgi regions from proximal ends of the cells into distal ends.

Clear cell free zone between the inner enamel epithelium and the dental papilla disappears.

The first appearance of dentin seems to be a critical phase in the life cycle of the inner enamel epithelium.

When dentin forms it cuts off the ameloblasts from their original source of nourishment.

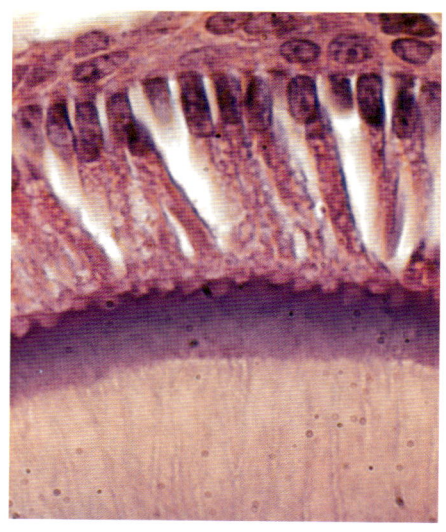

Fig. 3.8: Ameloblasts showing reverse functional polarity

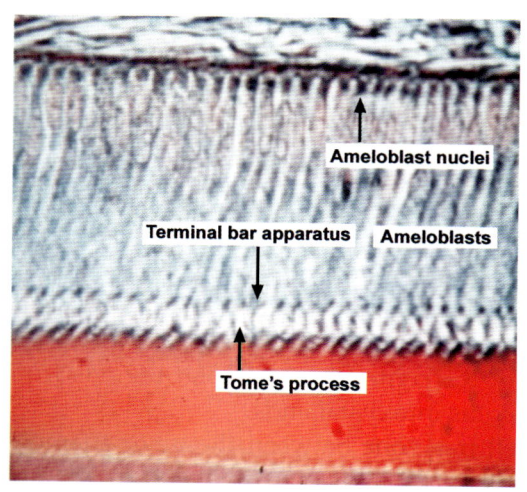

Fig. 3.9: Diagram showing reversal of polarity, Tome's process, terminal bar apparatus

The distance between the capillaries and the stratum intermedium and the ameloblast layer is shortened.

Enamel 39

FORMATIVE STAGE

The presence of dentin seems to be necessary for the beginning of enamel matrix formation.

This mutual interaction between one group of cells and another is one of the fundamental laws of organogenesis and histodifferentiation.

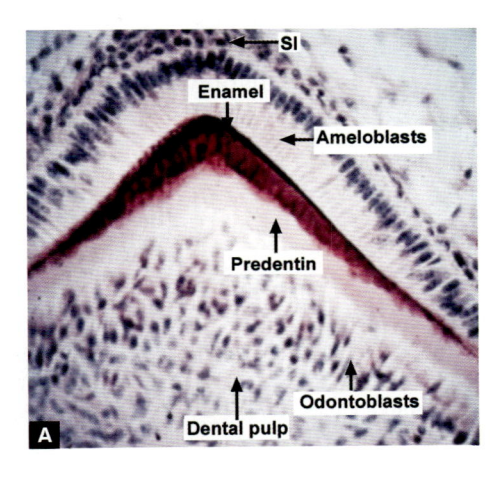

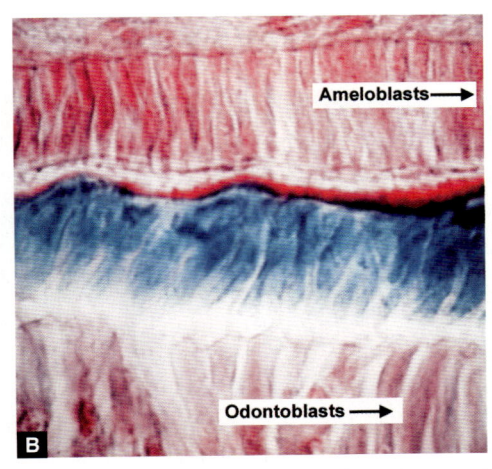

Figs 3.10A and B: Beginning of amelogenesis

The earliest apparent change is the development of blunt cell processes on the ameloblast surfaces, which penetrate the basal lamina and enter the predentin.

MATURATIVE STAGE

Occurs after most of the thickness of the enamel matrix has been formed in the occlusal or incisal area.

During enamel maturation the ameloblasts are slightly reduced in length. Cells of stratum intermedium assume a spindle shape. Ameloblasts display microvilli at their distal extremities, and cytoplasmic vacuoles.

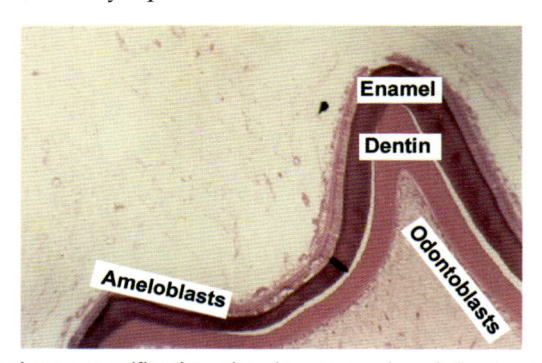

Fig. 3.11: Low magnification showing enamel and dentin deposition, ameloblast and odontoblast layer and dental papillae

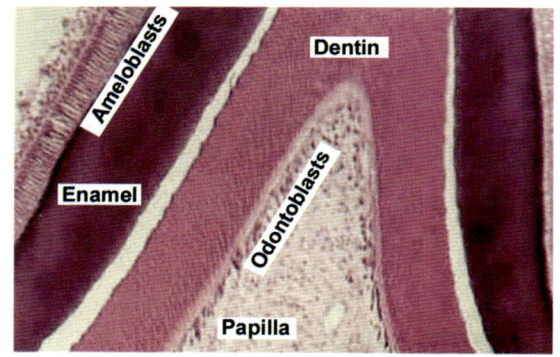

Fig. 3.12: A higher magnification showing ameloblasts, odontoblasts, enamel, dentin, and dental papilla

PROTECTIVE STAGE

The cell layers form a stratified epithelial covering of the enamel, the so called reduced enamel epithelium.

Its function is to protect the mature enamel by separating it from connective tissue until tooth erupts.

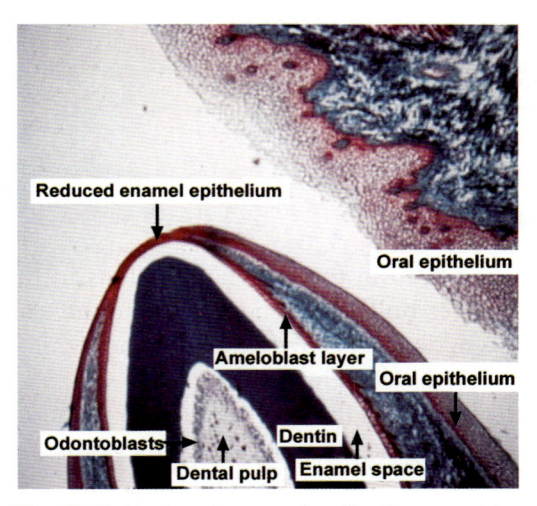

Fig. 3.13: Reduced enamel epithelium overlying the enamel of erupting tooth

If connective tissue comes in contact with enamel, anomalies may develop.

DESMOLYTIC STAGE

Reduced enamel epithelium proliferates and seems to induce atrophy of the connective tissue, separating it from oral epithelium, so that fusion of two epithelia can occur.

Epithelial cells elaborate enzymes that are able to destroy connective tissue fibers by desmolysis.

Premature degeneration of reduced enamel epithelium may prevent the eruption of a tooth.

Dentin

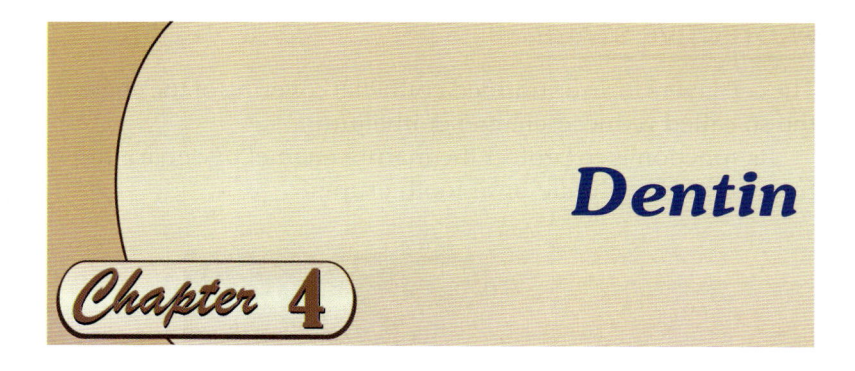

Chapter 4

INTRODUCTION

Dentin is found both in the crown as well as in the root and therefore provides bulk and general form to the teeth.

In the crown, dentin is covered by enamel while in the root dentin is covered by cementum.

Dentin determinates the morphology of the tooth.

It is a hard tissue which forms the bulk of the tooth.

It is the first formed hard tissue of the tooth.

Dentin and pulp are embryologically derived from the dental papilla.

PHYSICAL PROPERTIES

Color varies from light yellow in deciduous teeth to yellow in permanent dentition.

It is semitransparent.

It is less harder than enamel but more than bone or cementum.

It is less mineralized than enamel:
- It is highly elastic
- Modulus of elasticity is 1.6×10^7 psi
- Tensile strength is 6,000 psi
- Compressive strength is 40,000 psi

- It is highly permeable
- Permeability decreases with advancing age

  Shows positive birefringence under polarized light.

COMPOSITION

- Mature dentin contains   70% inorganic substance
  30% organic material and water
- Inorganic components   Hydroxyapatite
  Carbonate
  Trace elements
- Organic components   Predominantly collagen
  Small amount of citrate
  Chondroitin sulfate
  Protein
  Carbohydrate complexes

DEVELOPMENT (DENTINOGENESIS)

It is described in two stages:
1. Formation of matrix
2. Mineralization.

Formation of Matrix

Bundles of tropocollagen fibres are formed by subodontoblastic layer and they appear between the differentiating odontoblasts.

The fibrils spread out in a fan-like arrangement near the basement membrane.

The first formed dentin is known as mantle dentin.

Consists mainly of Korff's fibers and partly of fine network of collagenous fibrils having diameter of 0.05 mm.

These fine collagenous fibres predominate and Korff's fibres become less prominent.

These fine fibers are formed in the immediate vicinity of distal ends of odontoblasts.

Mineralization

After few microns of predentin is laid down mineralization of dentin starts near dentino-enamel junction in the form of small islands of globules that gradually fuse together and form a continuous layer of calcified dentin.

Earliest mineralization is in the form of fine hydroxyapatite crystals on the surface of collagen fibrils and ground substance.

Later crystals are laid down within fibrils themselves.

Formation and calcification of dentin begins at tips of the cusps or incisal edges and proceeds pulpally.

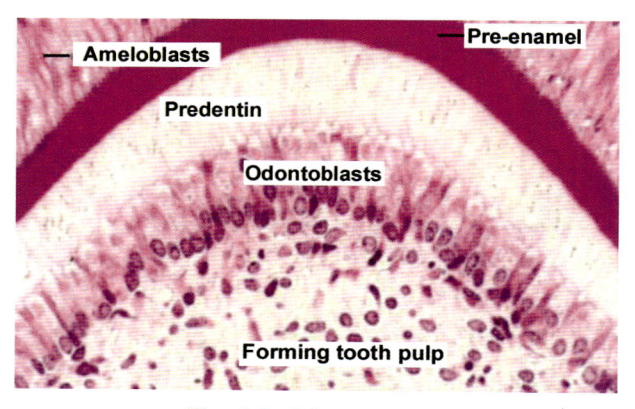

Fig. 4.1: Odontogenesis

STRUCTURES OF DENTIN

Dentinal Tubules

They are sigmoid shaped curved structures which run perpendicularly from the pulp towards periphery.

'S' shaped curves are primary curvatures.

The first curvature of these dentinal tubules is from the pulp towards the apex of the root.

Along the course small curvatures are seen which are called secondary curvatures.

Towards the pulp, the thickness varies from 2.5 to 4 µm thick.

Dentin 45

The dentinal tubules show branching and loop formation near the cementum. This area is seen as granular layer in ground sections and known as Tome's granular layer.

Contain odontoblastic processes which are filled with dentinal fluid

A thin organic sheath is found lining the dentinal tubules. This layer is called lamina limitans.

The odontoblastic process contains microfilaments, vesicles and ribosomes near the dentino-enamel junction.

Towards pulpal side they are rich in endoplasmic reticulum and mitochondria.

Odontoblastic cell bodies measure 7 µm in diameter and 40 µm in length.

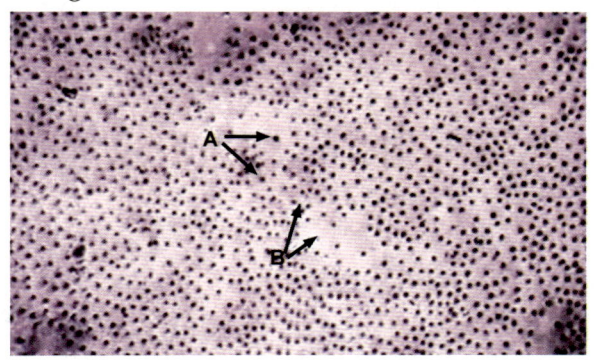

Fig. 4.2A: Dentinal tubules in cross-section

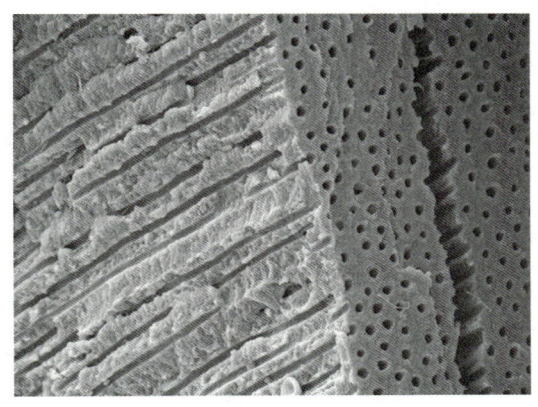

Fig. 4.2B: Electron microscopic view of dentinal tubules

Dentinoenamel Junction

Junction between enamel and dentin is irregular and is described as scalloped, having convexities facing the dentin whereas concavities facing the enamel.

Shape and nature of the junction by way of scalloping prevents shearing of the enamel during function.

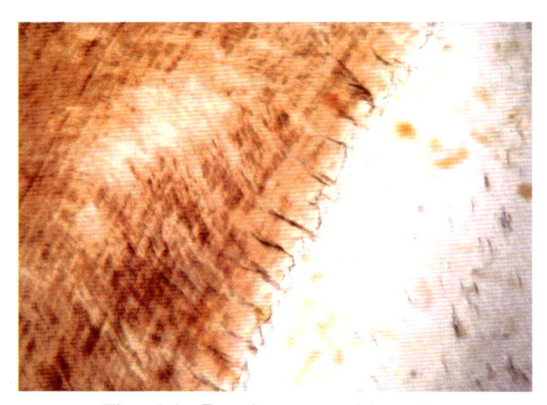

Fig. 4.3: Dentinoenamel junction

Intratubular (Peritubular Dentin)

Cross-section of the dentinal tubules when viewed in a ground section shows that dentinal tubules have hypermineralized area of dentin on their walls.

This dentin is called intratubular or peritubular dentin. This dentin is 44 µm wide near the DEJ.

It has more mineral content and less collagen.

When it obliterates several dentinal tubules, it forms sclerotic dentin.

Intertubular Dentin

It is present between the dentinal tubules.

Contains greater amount of organic matrix consisting of tightly interwoven network of type I collagen, phosphoproteins, proteoglycans, glucoproteins and plasma proteins.

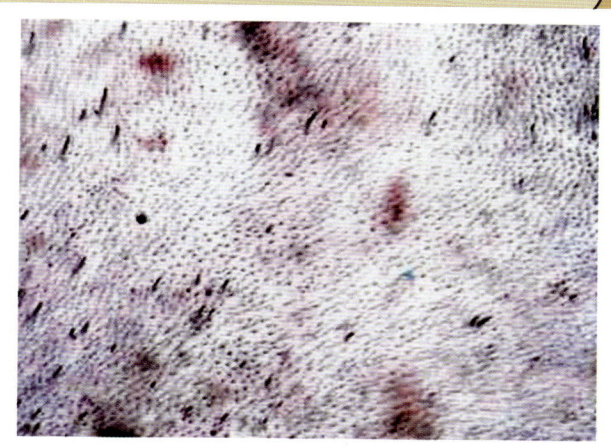

Fig. 4.4: Intertubular dentin

Mantle Dentin

First formed dentin present close to the dentinoenamel junction. It is less mineralized, 150 µm wide.

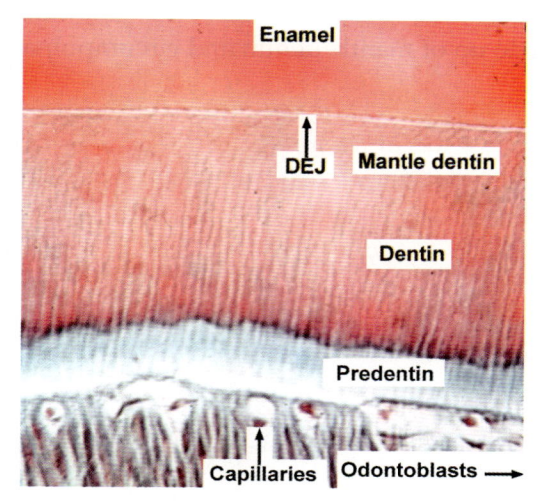

Fig. 4.5: Diagram showing various dentinal layers

Collagen fibers are arranged perpendicular to the dentino-enamel junction.

48 Oral Embryology and Histology

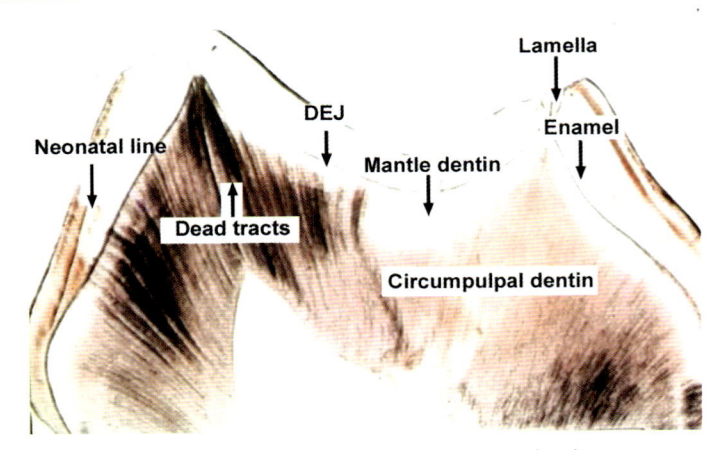

Fig. 4.6: Diagram showing primary dentin (Mantle dentin, circumpulpal dentin)

Primary Dentin

Forms the major bulk of dentin and is formed prior to root completion.
It is made up of mantle dentin and circumpulpal dentin.

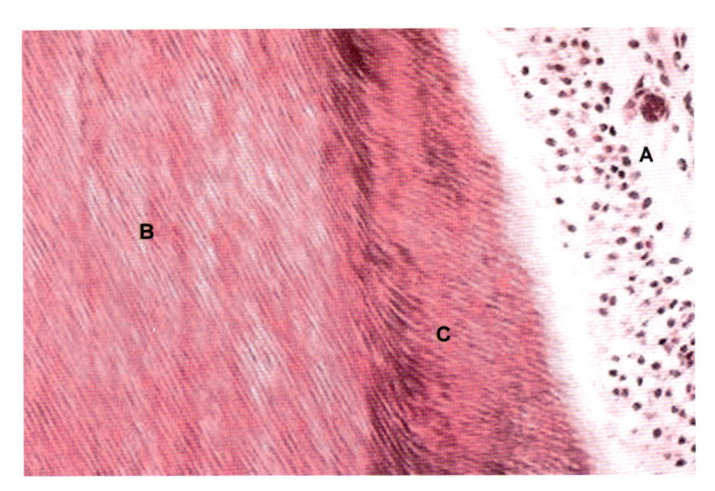

Fig. 4.7: (A) Pulp (B) Primary dentin (C) Secondary dentin

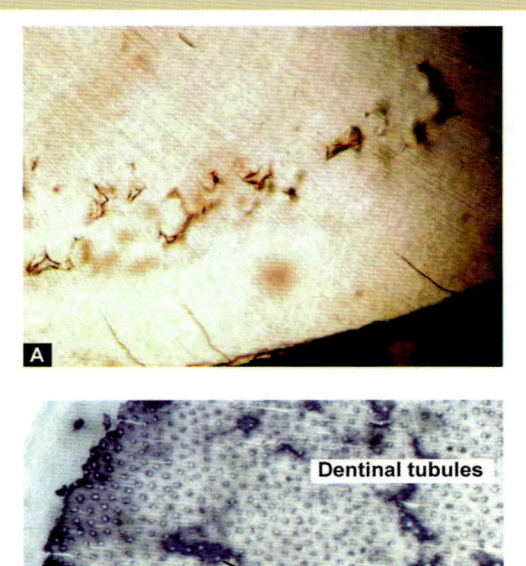

Figs 4.8A and B: Cross-section of tooth showing dentinal tubules and interglobular dentin

Circumpulpal Dentin

It is the primary dentin that surrounds the pulp.
  Better mineralized than mantle dentin.
  Collagen fibers are smaller in diameter, closely packed and parellel to the dentino-enamel junction.

Secondary Dentin

Narrow band of dentin adjacent to the pulp containing fewer tubules than primary dentin .
  Represents dentin formed after root completion.

Predentin

It is the innermost portion of dentin that is not mineralized and present adjacent to pulpal tissue.
 Represents the first formed dentin.
 Thickness 10-47 µm.
 As collagen fibers undergo mineralization, predentin gets converted to dentin and thus a new layer of predentin forms around the pulpal tissue.

Granular Layer of Tomes

Seen in ground sections of root dentin.
 Appears dark in transmitted light and lighter under reflected light.
 The amount increases from the CEJ to the apex of the root.
 Granular layer represents the looped terminal portion of the dentinal tubules in root dentin.
 Between Tomes' granular layer and cementum is found a structureless hyaline layer of 15 µm width. This layer is thought to be enameloid and is called layer of hopewell and smith.

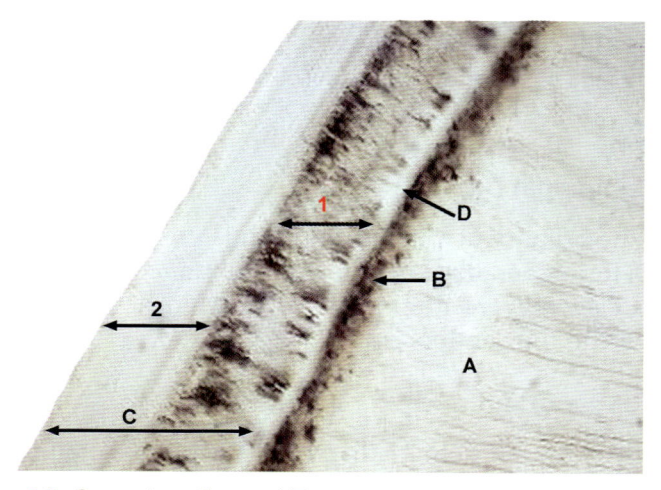

Fig. 4.9: Ground section and Tomes' granular layer (A) Dentin (B) Tomes' granular layer (C) Primary cementum (D) Hyaline layer

Dentin 51

STRUCTURAL LINES

One type of line is related to dentinogenesis and are called incremental lines (Lines of von Ebner).

The other type of lines are related to the curvature of the dentinal tubules (Contour lines of owen).

Incremental lines represent rhythmic activity of dentinogenesis.

Incremental Lines of von Ebner

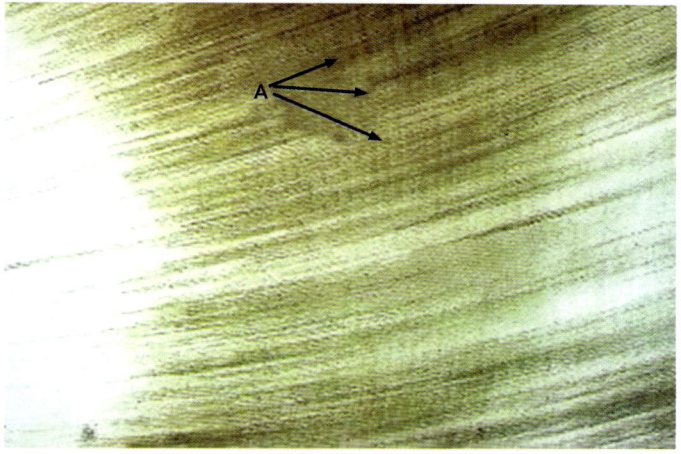

Fig. 4.10: (A) Incremental lines of von Ebner

Represent the 5 day rhythmic pattern of dentin deposition.

Mineralizing Lines

Represent variations in mineralization.

Seen in ground sections by microradiography or in demineralized sections.

Neonatal Line

It is a hypocalcified area represented by a wide contour line seen in those teeth that mineralize at birth.

For example: Deciduous dentition and first permanent molars.

Neonatal lines separates the dentin formed before and after birth.

Contour Lines of Owen

These lines result from coincidence of secondary curvatures between neighboring dentinal tubules.

Any accentuated hypomineralized line is known as contour line of owen.

A distinct contour line is seen at the junction of primary and secondary dentin.

AGE CHANGES IN DENTIN

1. Formation of secondary dentin
2. Dead tracts
3. Sclerotic dentin
4. Formation of reparative dentin (tertiary dentin).

Dead Tracts

These are dentinal tubules which appear dark under transmitted light and white under reflected light.

When tooth is subjected to external stimuli, the odontoblastic process may be lost in certain dentinal tubules.

These tubules are empty and are filled with air and appear dark in transmitted light.

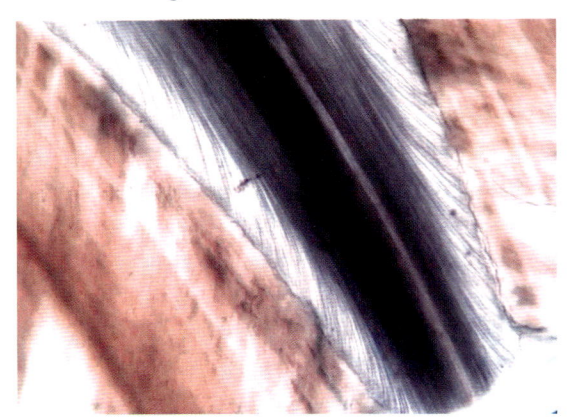

Fig. 4.11: Dead tracts

Sclerotic Dentin

Excessive formation of intratubular dentin can lead to complete obliteration of dentinal tubules.

When several tubules are obliterated they appear transparent.

Sclerotic dentin increases with age.

Mostly seen in apical third of root and in the crown midway between dentinoenamel junction and the pulpal surface.

Reparative Dentin

When odontoblasts die due to extensive erosion, abrasion, decay or operative procedures on the tooth, new odontoblasts are formed underlying pulpal undifferentiated perivascular cells.

Newly formed odontoblasts form reparative dentin to seal off the area so that inflammatory process is reduced.

Characterized by fewer tubules.

INNERVATION OF DENTIN

Contains numerous nerve endings in the predentin and inner dentin. These nerve endings are located in the tubules in the coronal zone, specifically in the pulp horns and interdigitate with the odontoblast process. The primary afferent somatosensory nerves of the dentin and pulp project to the decending trigeminal nuclear complex.

Three theories explaining dentin sensitivity.

Direct Nerve Stimulation Theory

Nerve endings in the dentin when stimulated, evoke a pain response.

Some nerves penetrate the dentinal tubules near the pulp.

Dentin sensitivity does not solely depend on nerve stimulation.

Hydrodynamic Theory

Dentinal tubules contain fluid called dental lymph.

The fluid movement through the dentinal tubules can disturb the pulp which is sensed by the plexus of Raschkow.

Tubules branch at DEJ, so there is increased sensitivity in this area.

Odontoblast Receptor Theory

Odontoblasts retain an ability to transduce and propagate to impulse.

Odontoblastic process are believed to extend to the DEJ.

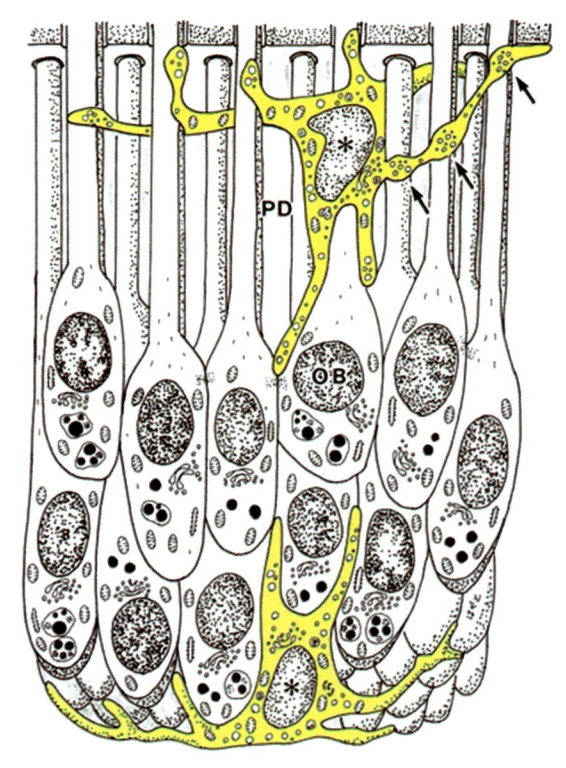

Fig. 4.12A: Diagram showing odontoblasts and dentinal tubules

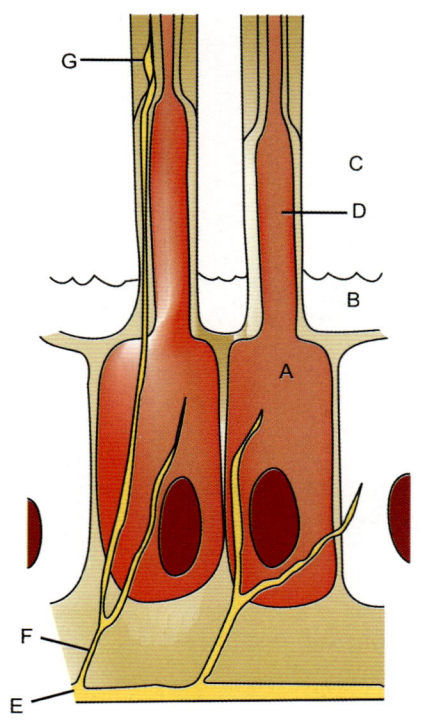

Fig. 4.12B: Illustrates the free nerve endings (F) arising from the subodontoblastic plexus (E) and passing up between odontoblasts (A) to enter the dentinal tubule where they terminate (G) on the odontoblast process (D) B = predentin, C = dentin

The gap junctions between odontoblasts or between odontoblasts and pulpal nerves can permit electron coupling.

Pulp

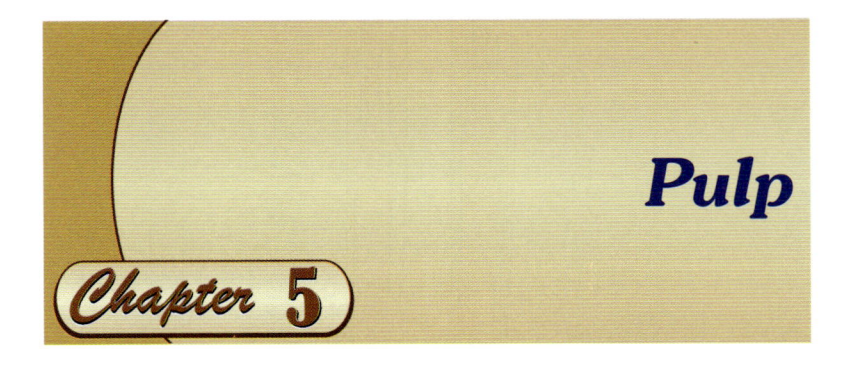

Chapter 5

DEFINITION

It is defined as a soft connective tissue which occupies the center of each tooth and supports the dentin.

ANATOMY

- Total number of pulp organs are 52.
    i. 32 permanent teeth
    ii. 20 primary teeth.
- Pulp organ conforms the same shape of the respective tooth.
- Total volume of all permanent pulp organs – 0.38 cc.
- Mean volume of adult human pulp – 0.02 cc.

MAXILLARY TEETH

Central Incisor

Shovel shaped, coronally tapering down to a triangle root in cross-section with the point of the triangle pointing lingually.

Lateral Incisor

Small spoon shaped coronally and becomes round evenly tapering root to the apex.

Cuspids

Longest pulp having elliptical in cross-section buccolingually and a distally inclined apex.

First Premolar

Large occluso-cervical pulp chamber with mesial concavity pulp chamber divides into two smooth funnel shaped root.

Second Premolar

Having one root which begins to taper at its midpoint.

Molars

Having a roughly rectangular cross-section with greatest dimension buccolingually and having mesiobuccal prominence, consists of 3 roots, lingual is the longest and distobuccal is shortest and straight. The mesiobuccal is curved and flattened buccolingually with its convex surface mesially.

MANDIBULAR TEETH

Central Incisor

One of the smallest pulp organ in the dentition and long narrow with flattened elliptical shape in cross-section buccolingually.

Lateral Incisor

Elliptical in cross-section and its root begins tapering at about its midpoint ending in a distally inclined apex.

Cuspids

It is similar to, but shorter than maxillary canine.

First Premolar

Features are similar to mandibular canine with an insignificant or missing lingual pulp horn.

Second Premolar

Same to mandibular canine with much smaller lingual horn than the buccal horn on the cervical region. It is triangular or some time rectangular.

Molars

Coronal cross-section is usually rectangular with mesiodistal dimension greatest with mesiobuccal prominence.

Pulp horns are mesio buccal, mesiolingual, distobuccal and distolingual.

Pulp organ is divided into 2 parts:
- Coronal pulp
- Radicular pulp.

Coronal Pulp

- Located centrally in the crown of teeth.
- It resembles the shape of the outer surface of the crown dentin.
- It consists of 6 surfaces:
  - Occlusal
  - Lingual
  - Distal
  - Buccal
  - Mesial
  - Floor
- Pulp horns are seen which are protrusions having extension into the cusps of each tooth.
- Number of horn depends on number of cusps.
- Cervical constriction is seen which follow the normal contour of the tooth.
- In this zone the coronal pulp joins the radicular pulp.

Radicular Pulp

- This extends from the cervical region of the crown to the root apex.
- In anteriors it is single and in posteriors it is multiple.
- It follows the normal contour of root of the tooth.

- Radicular pulp organ continues with periapical connective tissue through the apical foramen.
- The radicular pulp continues as apical pulp which becomes smaller because of apical cementum deposition.
- Basically pulp contains formative cells of dentin, defense cells for protection, undifferentiated mesenchymal cells, blood vessels and nerves. Macrophages and other immune component cells are also seen.

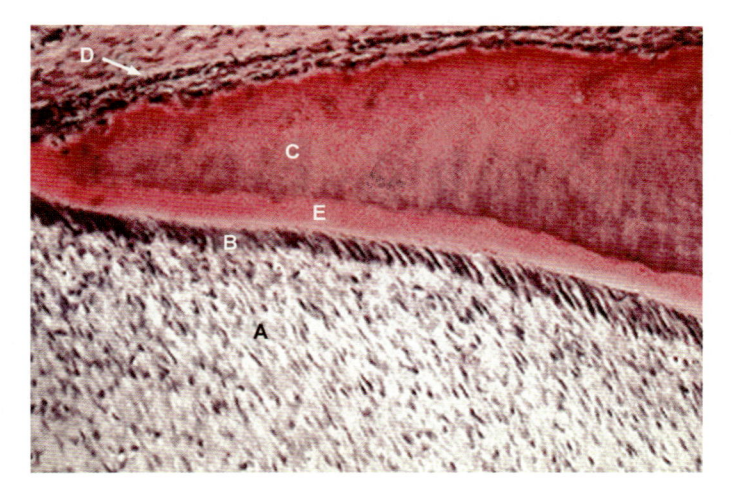

Fig. 5.1: Radicular pulp (A) Pulp (radicular) (B) Odontoblasts (C) Dentin (D) Epithelial root sheath (E) Predentin

STRUCTURAL FEATURES

On histological examination pulp consists of four zones:
- Odontoblastic zone
- Cell free zone
- Cell rich zone
- Pulp core.

Odontoblastic zone is the peripheral zone which contains dentin forming cells. Cell free zone, also called as zone of Weil or Weil's basal layer, seen beneath the odontoblasts which is

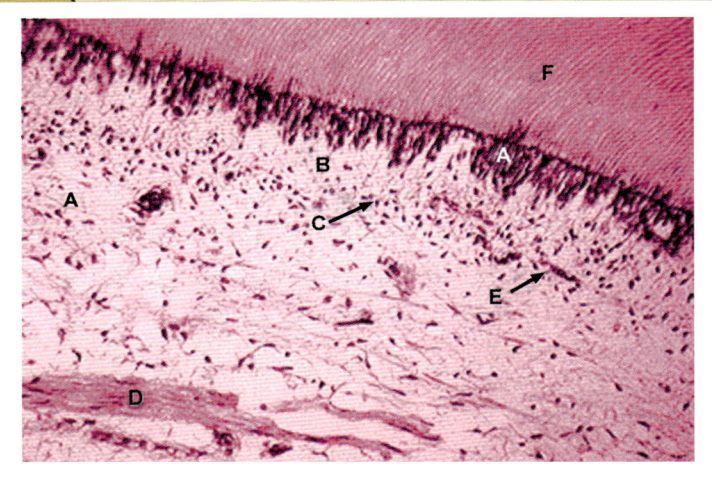

Fig. 5.2: Zones of pulp (A) Odontoblast layer (B) Cell-free zone (C) Cell-rich zone (D) Nerve pleus (E) Capillary (F) Dentin

prominent in the coronal pulp. Cell rich zone is an area of pulpal tissue where cell density is high mainly seen in coronal pulp adjacent to the cell-free zone. This layer is mainly composed of fibroblasts and undifferentiated mesenchymal cells. Pulp core characterized by the presence of major vessels and nerves.

Odontoblasts

Most distinctive cells of the dental pulp, so most easily recognized (second most prominent cell).

These cells form a single layer lining the periphery of the pulp and have a process extending into the dentin.

In the crown portion, odontoblasts often appear to be arranged in a palisading pattern seemingly forming a layer about 3-5 cells in depth.

The number of odontoblasts has been estimated to be in the range of 45,000/- sq mm in coronal dentin with a lesser number in root dentin.

5-7 mm in diameter and 25-40 mm in length.

Coronal portion	Radicular portion
• Arranged in a palisading arrangement • 3-5 layers of cells are seen • No. of odontoblasts estimated as 45,000/sq.mm • Length is larger • Cell body is columnar-shaped	• No definite arrangement only 1-2 layers seen • No. of odontoblasts estimated as 10-15,000/sq mm • Length is smaller • Cell body is cuboidal to flattened-shaped

Cells show a pseudostratified arrangement due to crowding.

According to morphology odontoblasts are classified in four stages:
  i. Preodontoblasts
  ii. Secretory
  iii. Transitional
  iv. Aged

These stages reflect the functional activity of the cell.

The organelles of an active odontoblast are prominent consisting of numerous vesicles, much endoplasmic reticulum, a well-developed Golgi complex located on the dentinal side of the nucleus and numerous mitochondria scattered throughout the cell body.

Odontoblastic process begins at the neck of the odontoblast, where the cell gradually begins to narrow in diameter as it passes through the predentin into mineralized dentin.

These odontoblasts maintain some complex junctions between each other. It is ia combination of:
  a. Gap junctions
  b. Zonula occludens (tight junction)
  c. Zonula adherence (desmosomes).

Occurrence of gap junction between adjacent odontoblast indicates communication between these cells.

Intercellular Substances

It is dense and gel like in nature, varies in appearance from finely granular to fibrillar.

It is composed of mucopolysacchrides and protein polysaccharide compounds, i.e. glycosoaminoglycans and proteoglycans.

During early development presence of chondroitin 'A' 'B' and hyaluronic acid is seen, glycoproteins are also seen.

Function

Support the cells of the pulp and it serves as a means of transport of nutrients from the blood vessels to the cells as well as for transport of metabolites from cells to blood vessels.

Fibroblast

- Cells occurring in the greatest number.
- Particularly numerous in the coronal portion where they form cell rich zone.
- Characterized by typical stellate shape and extensive processes of other fibroblasts.
- In the young pulp the cells divide and are active in protein synthesis. But in older pulp they appear rounded or spindle shaped with short processes called "Fibrocytes."

Function

- Helps in collagen fiber formation throughout the pulp.
- To form and maintain the pulp matrix which consists of collagen and ground substance.

Undifferentiated Mesenchymal Cells

- Primary cells seen in the very young pulp that may be seen after root completion.
- Appears larger than the fibroblast and are polyhedral in shape with peripheral processes and large oval nuclei.

- Found along pulp vessels in the cell rich zone and scattered throughtout the central pulp.
- They are believed to be totipotent cell and when needed they may become odontoblast, fibroblasts or macrophages.
- Decrease in number in old age.

Defense Cells

This consists of histiocytes, macrophages, mast cells and plasma cells.

In addition, there are blood vascular elements such as the neutrophils, eosinophils, basophils, lymphocytes and monocytes.

Macrophage has perivascular distribution and appears as a large oval or spindle shaped cell, exhibits a dark staining cytoplasm and darker nucleus.

Functions

Helps in elimination of dead cells which indicates turnover in the dental pulp.

When inflammation occurs the macrophage, it removes bacteria and interacts with other inflammatory cells.

Lymphocyte also called lymphoid cells is another cell mostly shows a focal accumulation in unerupted and newly erupted teeth.

T-Lymphocytes are mainly found having same function to Langerhans' cell.

BLOOD VESSELS OF PULP

- Pulp organ is extensively vascularized.
- Pulp and periodontium is mainly supplied by inferior or superior alveolar artery and drain by the same veins in both mandibular and maxillary region.
- Some vascularization is also seen through accessory canals.
- Blood vessels enter and exist the dental pulp by apical and accessory foramen.

- In the coronal region of the pulp they divide and subdivide to form an extensive vascular capillary network.
- Occasionally 'U' looping of pulpal arterioles is seen and this anatomic configuration is thought to be related to the regulation of blood flow.
- The flow of the blood in arterioles is 0.3-1 mm/sec.
- In venules it may be 0.15 mm/sec.
- In capillaries it may be 0.08 mm/sec.
- Largest arteries in the human pulp are 50-100 mm in diameter, thus equalizing in size of the arterioles found in most areas of the body.
- Occasionally a fibroblast or pericyte lie on the surface of these vessels.

Pericytes

These are capillary associated fibroblasts and their nuclei can be distinguished as round or slightly oval bodies closely associated with the outer surface of the terminal arterioles or precapillaries.

Also called as *"Rouget s cells"*. Both venous—venous anastomoses and arteriovenous anastomoses occur in the pulp. Arterio-venous shunt may have an important role in regulation of pulpal blood flow.

Functions of Pericytes

Still controversial but it is thought that they serve as contractile cell capable of reducing the size of the vessel lumen.

Lymphatic vessels are small, thin walled vessels in the coronal region of the pulp and differentiated from small venules by absence of RBC in their lumen.

This circulation establishes the tissue fluid pressure found in the extracellular compartment of the pulp.

Circulation of the volume of this fluid in the coronal portion of the tooth indicate that it constitutes about 20% of volume of dentin near the pulp and 4% near the enamel.

Mean volume of fluid in dentin is 10%.

Alteration of fluid produces clinical symptom of pain.

Lymph vessels draining the pulp and periodontal ligament have a common outlet.

Those draining the anterior teeth pass to the submental lymph nodes and posterior teeth pass to submandibular and deep cervical lymph nodes.

NERVE SUPPLY OF PULP

Innervation accompanies the blood vessels which together form the neurovascular bundle.

It has been estimated that each nerve fiber may provide at least eight terminal branches which ultimately contribute to an extensive plexus of nerves in the cell free zone just below the cell bodies of the odontoblasts in the crown portion of the tooth. This is called as *subodontoblastic plexus* or *"plexus of Raschkow."*

Nerve fibers are sensory afferent of the trigeminal (5th) and sympathetic branches from the superior cervical ganglion.

Each bundle contains both myelinated and unmyelinated axons.

These are classified according to their diameter and conduction velocities.
   i. Majority are a fiber → diameter → 1-6 mm.
   ii. 1% is a beta → diameter → 6-12 mm.
   iii. Nonmyelinated fibers are designated as 'C' fibers having → diameter → 1.4-1.2 mm.

A alpha → Sharp localized pain experienced when dentin is first exposed.

C → Dull diffuse pain.

A beta → Mechanical thermal and tactile receptors also exist.

Most of the nerve bundles terminate in the subodontoblastic plexus as free nerve endings.

A small number of axons loose their Schwann cell coating and pass between the odontoblast cell bodies to enter the dentinal tubules in close approximation to the odontoblastic process.

FUNCTIONS OF THE PULP

Functions are:
  i. *Inductive:* Pulp induces oral epithelial differentiation into dental lamina and enamel organ formation and also induce the developing enamel organ to become a particular type of tooth.
  ii. *Formative:* Helps in production of dentin.
  iii. *Nutritive:* Pulp nourishes the dentin through the odontoblasts blood vessels.
  iv. *Protective:* Helps in protection from heat, cold, pressure, operative cutting procedures and chemical agents by producing stimuli called pain.
  v. *Defensive or reparative:* It responds to irritation. It may be mechanical, thermal, chemical or bacterial by producing reparative dentin and mineralizing any affected dentinal tubules.

REGRESSIVE CHANGES OF PULP

A. *Cell changes*
  – Decrease in size and number of cytoplasmic organelles.
  – Fibroblasts exhibit less perinuclear cytoplasm and possess long thin cytoplasmic processes.
  – Intracellular organelles are reduced in number and size.
B. *Fibrosis*
  – Accumulation of both diffuse fibrillar components as well as bundles of collagen fibers usually appear.
  – Small amount of collagen accumulation seen.
C. *Pulp stones (denticles)* are frequently found in pulp tissue
  • Characterized by discrete calcified masses which are nodular in mass.
  • May be seen in coronal or radicular part.

Classification

a. *According to their structure:*
  i. *True denticles:* Similar to dentin, rarely seen and usually located at apical foramen.

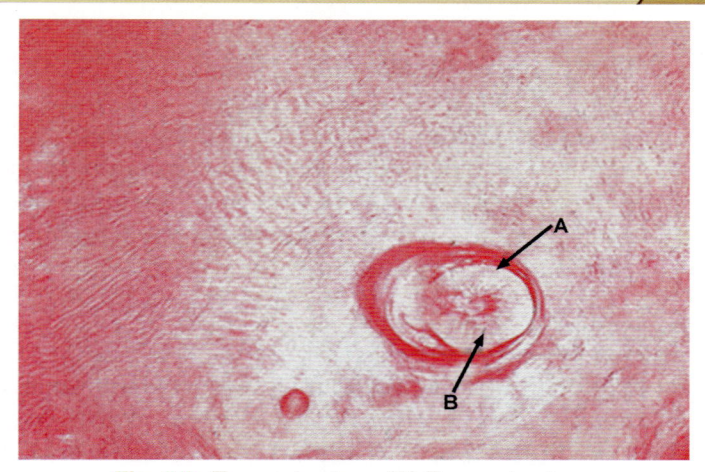

Fig. 5.3: True pulp stone (A) True pulp stone (B) Dentinal tubules

ii. *False denticles:* It is caused by the inclusion of remnants of epithelial root sheath within pulp. They do not contain dentinal tubules.

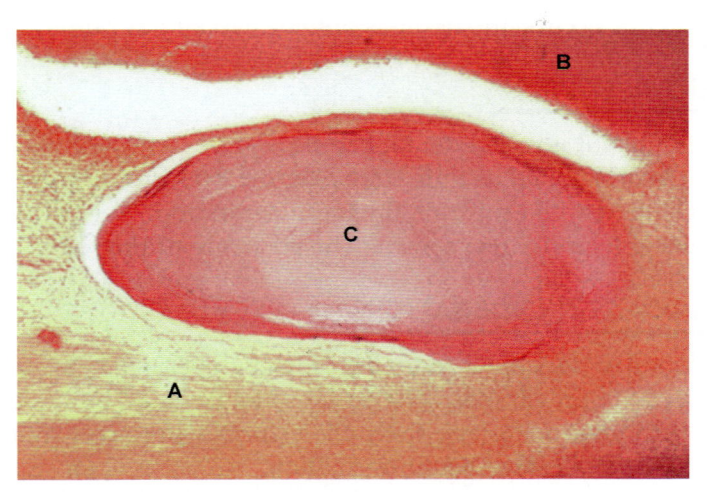

Fig. 5.4: False pulp stones (A) Pulp (B) Dentin (C) False pulp stone

iii. Diffuse denticles.

b. *According to their location:*
   i. *Free:* Lying free in the pulp.
   ii. *Attached:* Attached to dentin.
   iii. *Embedded:* Completely surrounded by dentin. If it is entraped on blood vessel, nerve then it may cause pain.
   iv. *Diffuse calcification:* These appear as irregular calcification deposits in the pulp tissue usually found in root canal and less often in the coronal area.

DEVELOPMENT OF PULP

Dental papilla proliferates at about 8th week of embryonic life in the human.

Cells of dental papilla appears as undifferentiated mesenchymal cells.

Gradually these cells differentiate into stellate shaped fibroblasts.

After the inner enamel organ cells differentiate into ameloblasts, the odontoblasts then differentiate from the peripheral cells of the dental papilla and dentin production begins.

As this occurs, the tissue is now designated as pulp organ.

DENTAL PAPILLA

- Initially it is called dental papilla.
- It is designated as pulp only after dentin forms around it.
- Dental papilla **controls the tooth formation.**
- Dental papilla also controls **the structure of the tooth.**

CLINICAL CONSIDERATIONS

In young or deciduous tooth the pulp chamber will be wide, so deep cavity preparation is hazardous and it should be avoided.

With advancing age the pulp chamber becomes smaller because of excessive dentin formation.

When accessory canals are located near the coronal part of the root or in the bifurcation area, a deep periodontal pocket may cause inflammation of the dental pulp.

Thus, periodontal disease can have a profound influence on pulp integrity.

A necrotic pulp can cause spread of disease to periodontium through an accessory canal.

It is recognized that pulpal and periodontal disease may spread by their common blood supply.

Exposed pulps can be preserved if proper capping procedures are applied unless it is uninfected.

A severe reaction in pulp is characterized by one with increased inflammatory cells infiltration adjacent to the cavity site which leads to hyperemia or localized abscess.

Usually the closer a restoration is to the pulp organ the greater will be the pulp response.

A nonvital tooth becomes brittle and is subject to fracture.

Vitality of the pulp depends upon the blood supply.

One can have teeth with damaged nerve but normal blood supply. Such pulps don't respond to electrical or thermal stimuli but are completely viable in every respect.

Cementum (Substantia Ossea)

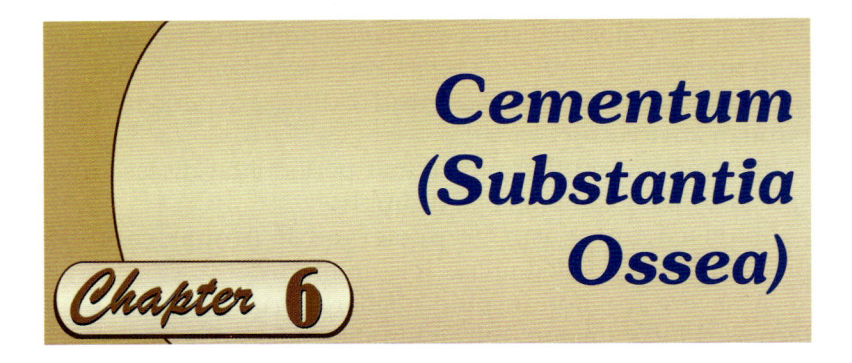

Chapter 6

INTRODUCTION

Cementum is the mineralized dental tissue covering the roots of human teeth.

It furnishes a medium for the attachment of collagen fibers that bind the tooth to the surrounding structure.

It is avascular. Thus, it exhibits increased resistance to resorption.

Physical Characteristics

- Light yellow in color.
- Hardness is less than that of dentin.
- Cementum is thinnest at CEJ (20-50 nm) and thickest towards apex (150 to 200 nm).

Chemical Composition

- 45 to 50%—Inorganic substances
  - Calcium hydroxyapatite
  - Phosphate hydroxyapatite

- 50 to 55%—Organic material and water
  - Type I collagen
  - Protein polysaccharides

- Cementum has the highest fluoride content.

Cementogenesis

Cementum formation is preceded by the deposition of dentin along the inner aspect of Hertwig's epithelial root sheath.

Once dentin formation begins, break occurs along the Hertwig's epithelial root sheath allowing the newly formed dentin to come in direct contact with the connective tissue of the dental follicle.

Cells derived from this connective tissue (cementoblasts) are responsible for cementum formation.

(Some sheath cells that migrate towards the dental sac become the epithelial rests of malassez found in the Periodontal Ligament).

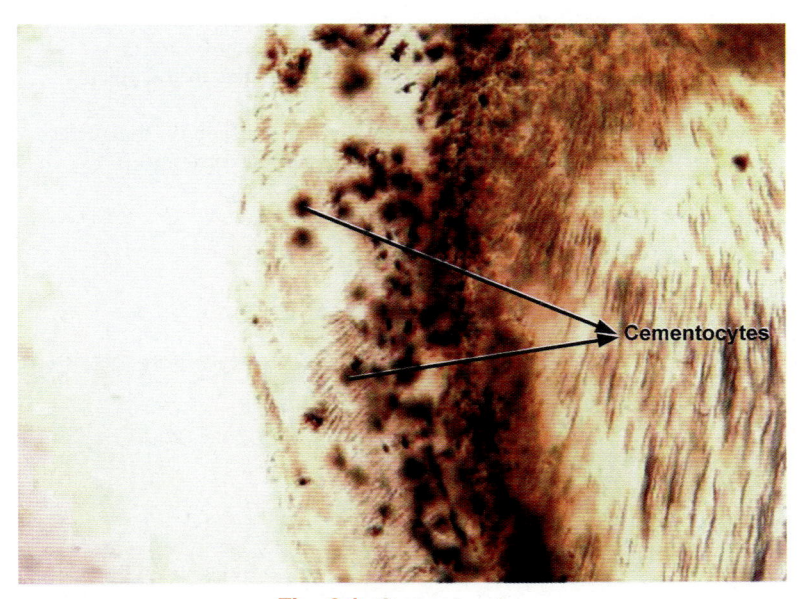

Fig. 6.1: Cementocytes

Cementoblasts

Derived from the undifferentiated mesenchymal cells of the adjacent connective tissue (dental sac).

Cementoid

The uncalcified matrix of cementum is called cementoid. It is lined by cementoblasts. Connective tissue fibers from the Periodontal ligament are embedded in the cementum and serve to attach tooth to surrounding bone (Bundle bone). These embedded fibers are known as Sharpey's fibers.

Structure

- Cementum
  - Acellular
  - Cellular

Acellular	Cellular
• Devoid of cementoblast	• Cementoblasts are seen
• Covers the root from CEJ to the apex	• Seen in apical 3rd of root
• Predominates in the coronal half of the root	• Predominates in the apical half of root
• Occasionally found on the surface of cellular cementum	• Frequently seen on the surface of acellular cementum

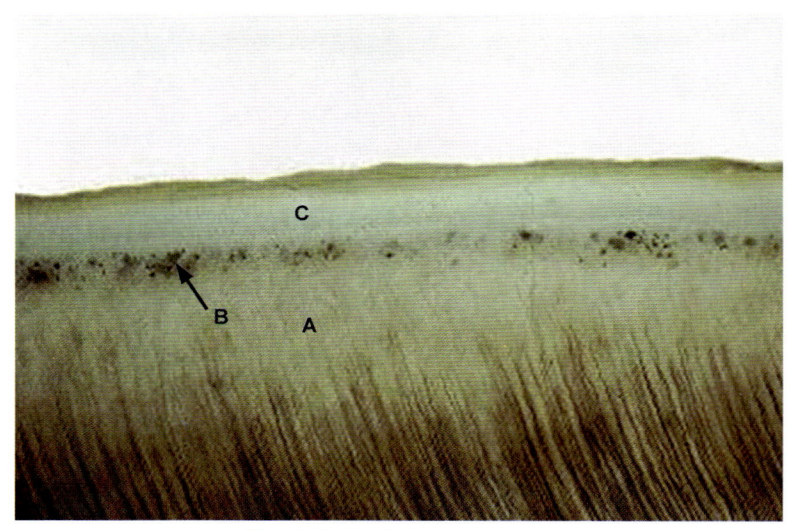

Fig. 6.2: Acellular cementum
(A) Dentin (B) Tomes' granular layer (C) Primary cementum

Cementum (Substantia Ossea) 73

Both acellular and cellular cementum are separated by incremental lines (Incremental lines of Salter) into layers, which indicate periodic formation. They are highly mineralized areas with less collagen.

Cementodentinal Junction

In deciduous teeth the cemento-dentinal junction is seen as scalloped line. In permanent teeth it is seen as smooth line.

The interface between cementum and dentin is clearly visible in decalcified and stained histological sections.

Sometimes dentin is separated from cementum by a zone known as the intermediate cementum layer. The layer is predominantly seen in the apical 2/3rd of roots of molars and premolars. This layer represents areas where cells of Hertwig's epithelial root sheath become trapped in a rapidly deposited dentin or cementum matrix. Intermediate cementum is rarely seen in deciduous teeth and anterior teeth.

Cementoenamel Junction

30% of teeth — Cementum meets the cervical end of enamel in a relatively sharp line.

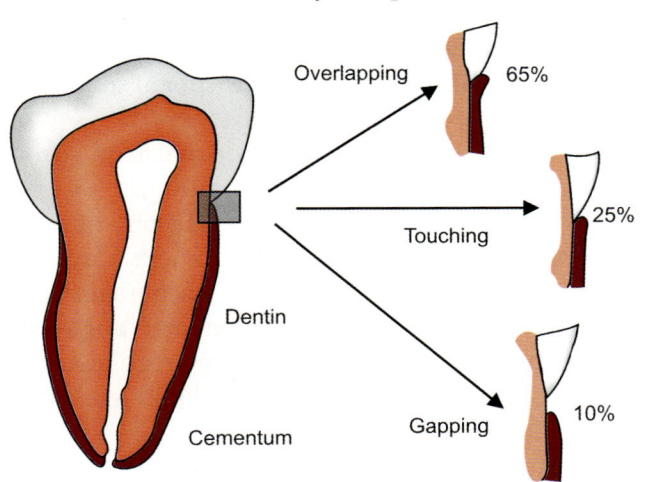

Fig. 6.3: Types of cementoenamel junction

10% of teeth – Enamel and dentin do not meet.
60% of teeth – Cementum overlaps the cervical end of enamel for a short distance.

Cementoblasts contacts enamel surface produce afibrillar cementum. Afibrillar cementum contacts connective tissue cells and forms fibrillar cementum (Afibrillar devoid of fibrils of 640 Å periodicity).

Function

Furnish a medium for the attachment of collagen fibers that bind the tooth to alveolar bone.

Continuous deposition of cementum is of functional importance. As the superficial layer of cementum ages, a new layer must be deposited to keep the attachment intact.

It is the major reparative tissue for root surfaces damage to roots such as fractures and resorptions can be repaired by the deposition of new cementum.

Hypercementosis

- Abnormal thickening of cementum.
- May be diffuse of circumscribed.
- May affect all teeth or single tooth.
- If the overgrowth improves the functional qualities of the cementum-cementum hypertrophy.
- If the overgrowth occurs in non-functional teeth – cementum hyperplasia.
- If teeth exposed to great stress, hypertrophy of cementum forms prong like extensions, which provides a larger surface area for the attaching fibers – firmer anchorage.
- Hyperplastic cementum covers the enamel drops which are found on the dentinal surface. They are irregular and contain round calcified epithelial rests. Such knob like projections are termed excementoses.
- Cementum is thicker around the apex of all teeth and in the furcation of multirooted teeth.

Clinical Considerations

Cementum is more resistant to resorption than bone because cementum is avascular; bone is vascular.

Cemental resorption is repaired by formation of cellular or acellular cementum or by both. This is called anatomic repair.

Thin layer of cementum is deposited on the surface of a deep resorption and a bay-like recess remains. In such areas, the periodontal space is restored to its normal width by formation of a bony projection, so that proper functional relationship is maintained. This is called functional repair.

Periodontal Ligament

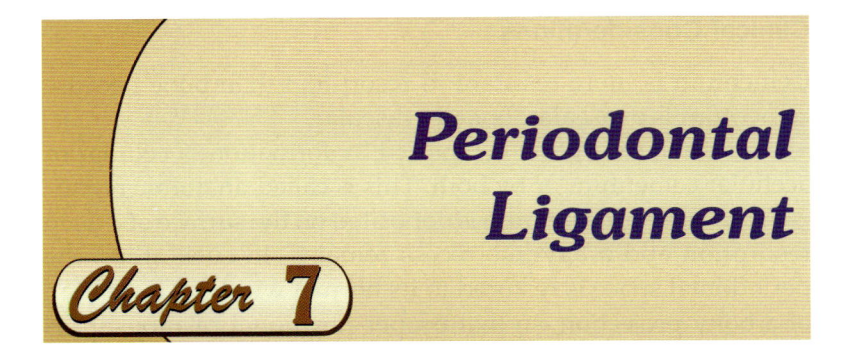

Chapter 7

The periodontal ligament is a specialized connective tissue which surrounds the root of tooth, occupying the space between the root and the alveolar bone of tooth socket.

The periodontal ligament is also called periodontal membrane.

It ranges in width from 0.15-0.38 mm with the thinnest portion at the middle third of root.

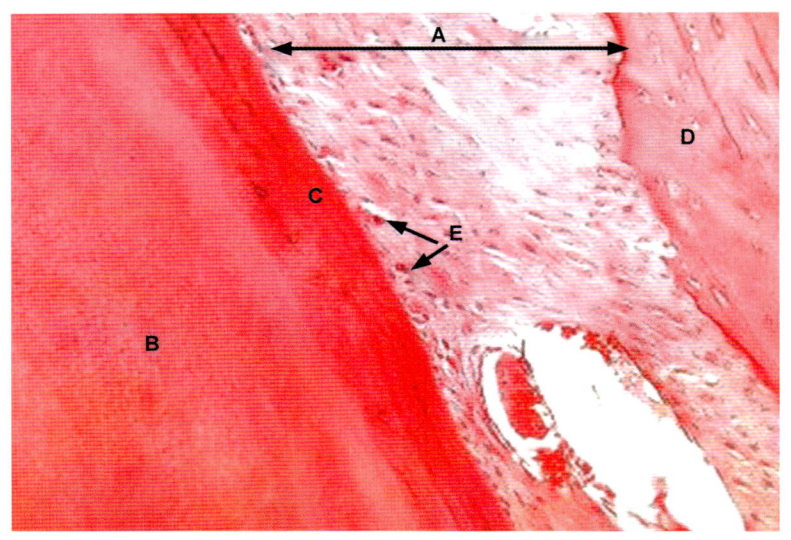

Fig. 7.1: (A) Periodontal ligament (B) Dentin (C) Cementum (D) Alveolar bone (E) Epithelial rests

Periodontal Ligament

On an average it is 0.21 mm in width.

It shows progressive decrease in its width with age, by about 50 years its width reduces to as much as 0.15 mm.

DEVELOPMENT OF PERIODONTAL LIGAMENT

The enamel organ is surrounded by condensation of mesenchymal cells called the dental sac.

The part of dental sac immediately close to enamel organ is called the dental follicle.

The part of dental sac that surrounds the dental follicle is called perifollicular mesenchyme.

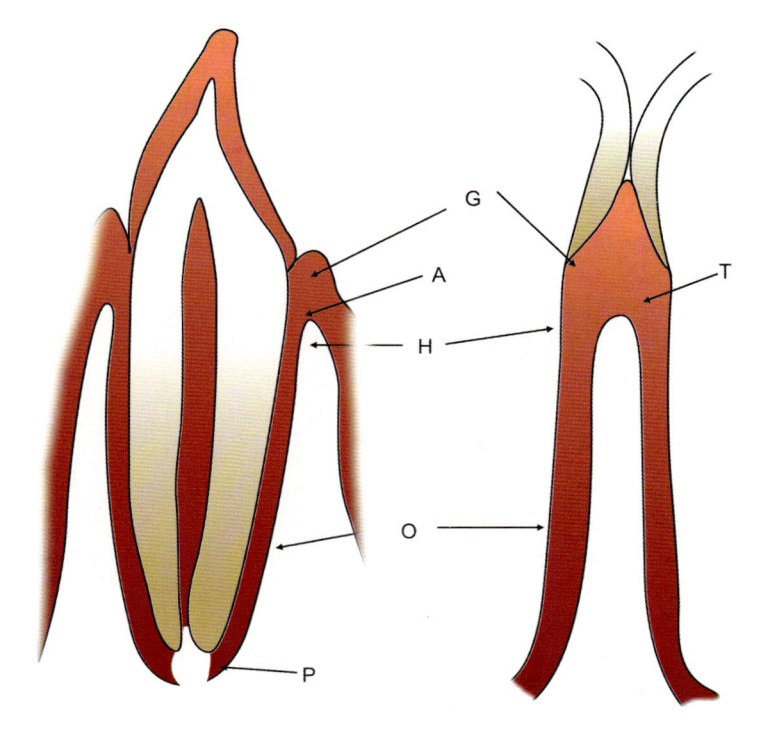

Fig. 7.2: Principal fibers of periodontal ligament (A) Alveolar crest fibers (G) Gingival fibers (H) Horizontal fibers (O) Oblique fibers (P) (Periapical fibers (T) Trans-septal fibers

Once Hertwig's epithelial root sheath disintegrates leaving behind the epithelial rests of Malassez, cells of dental follicle come close to surface of newly formed dentin.

The dental follicle cells differentiate into cementoblasts and lay down cementum on dentin.

The other cells of dental follicle differentiate into fibroblasts and lay down periodontal ligament.

FUNCTIONS OF PERIODONTAL LIGAMENT

It has 5 important functions:

Supportive

Whenever a tooth is moved in its socket, the ligament gets compressed and provides support for the tooth.

The collagen fibers that occur in periodontal ligament act as a cushion to withstand force.

The fibers are so arranged that functional pressure on teeth from any direction produces tension on certain fibers, therefore pressure on tooth crown is transmitted to the bone of tooth socket.

The ground substance present between the fibers of periodontal ligament is rich in water content and therefore add up to the support.

Formative

During the development of tooth, the cells of ligament produce cementum and bone of tooth socket.

The ligament contains cementoblasts and osteoblasts that can form new cementum and bone respectively.

Resorptive

Pressure on periodontal ligament tends to cause bone resorption.

The resorptive processes are brought about by osteoclast cells present in periodontal ligament.

Sensory

Periodontal ligament provides an excellent proprioceptive mechanism which helps in estimating the amount of pressure on mastication and elicits even the mildest force acting upon a tooth.

Nutritive

The periodontal ligament has a good blood supply which provides nutrition for cells.

Whenever very heavy forces are applied on tooth the periodontal ligament may necrose.

STRUCTURE OF PERIODONTAL LIGAMENT

Periodontal ligament consists of cells, ground substance, fibers and other structures such as blood vessels and nerves.

a. Cells of Periodontal Ligament

Synthetic cells	Resorbing cells
Osteoblasts	Osteoclasts
Fibroblasts	
Cementoblasts	Cementoclasts

Other Cells

Epithelial cell rests of malassez, mast cells and macrophages.

Osteoblasts

They are bone forming cells that are derived from multipotent mesenchymal cells.

They have prominent Golgi apparatus, mitochondria and rough endoplasmic reticulum.

Fibroblasts

They help in resorption and synthesis of extracellular connective tissue.

They are usually found parallel to collagen fibers.

Cementoblasts

They help in formation of cementum.

Osteoclasts

They are bone resorbing cells that are large and generally occur in clusters.

An increase in number of osteoclasts are seen where bone is undergoing active resorption.

Cementoclasts

As cementum does not remodel these cells are not normally found in ligament.

These cells occur only in certain pathologic conditions, during resorption of deciduous teeth and during orthodontic therapy.

Other Cells

Mast cells and macrophages that are derived from monocytes are present in ligament.

Epithelial Cells of Malassez

These cells may be found in ligament close to cemental surface.

These are remnants of Hertwig's epithelial root sheath.

b. Fibers of Periodontal Ligament

1. Collagen fibers.
2. Oxytalan fibers.

Collagen Fibers

Collagen fibers of periodontal ligament is a mixture of type I and III.

The bundles of collagen fibers are arranged in groups having a clear orientation in periodontal spaces.

These fiber groups are called principle fibers.

They are arranged in five distinct groups.

Alveolar Crest Group

These fibers are attached to cementum below cementoenamel junction. They run downwards and outwards to insert into alveolar crest.

Horizontal Group

They are found apical to alveolar crest group. They run at right angles from cementum to alveolar bone.

Oblique Group

They run from cementum to bone in oblique direction. They are the most numerous fibers seen.

Apical Group

They run from cementum to root apex.

Inter-radicular Group

They run from furcation area of multirooted tooth to crest of inter-radicular septum.

Oxytalan Fibers

Oxytalan fibers are elastic fibers that tends to run in any direction. One end is attached to cementum or alveolar bone while the other end gets attached to blood vessels. Thus, they support the periodontal ligament blood vessels.

Ground Substance

- It is made up of proteins and polysaccharides which are proteoglycans and glycoproteins.
- It contains about 70% water.
- The ground substance helps in transporting food to cells and also helps in carrying the waste products from cells to blood vessels.

OTHER STRUCTURES IN PERIODONTAL LIGAMENT

Blood Vessels

The blood vessels of periodontal ligament is derived from:
- Gingival vessels
- Intra-alveolar vessels
- Vessels that supplies pulp.

Nerves

The nerves are derived from second and third division of trigeminal nerve (5th). The nerve fibers are large myelinated and small nonmyelinated fibers.

Alveolar Process

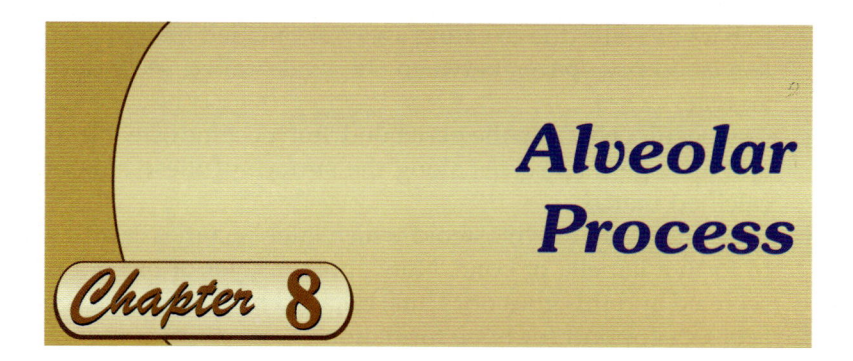

Chapter 8

DEVELOPMENT

Bone formation takes place in two ways.
1. Endochondral bone formation.
2. Intramembranous bone formation.

ENDOCHONDRAL BONE FORMATION

Bone formation is preceded by formation of a cartilaginous model which is subsequently replaced by bone.

Occurs as follows:
a. Mesenchymal cells become condensed at the site of bone formation.
b. Mesenchymal cells differentiate into chondroblasts and lay down hyaline cartilage.
c. Cartilage is surrounded by a membrane called perichondrium. This is highly vascular and contains osteogenic cells.
d. Intercellular substance becomes calcified due to the influence of enzyme alkaline phosphatase secreted by the cartilage cells.
e. Nutrition to the cartilage cells is cut off leading to death. This results in formation of empty spaces called primary areolae.
f. Blood vessels and osteogenic cells from the perichondrium invade calcified cartilagenous matrix which is now reduced

to bars or walls due to eating away of calcified matrix. This leaves empty spaces between the walls called secondary areolae.

g. Osteogenic cells from the perichondrium become osteoblasts and arrange themselves along the surface of these bars of calcified matrix.
h. Osteoblasts lay down osteoid which later becomes calcified to form a lamella of bone. Now another layer of osteoid is secreted and this goes on. Thus, calcified matrix of cartilage acts as a support for bone formation.

INTRAMEMBRANOUS BONE FORMATION

Formation of bone is not preceded by formation of a cartilagenous model.

Instead bone is laid down directly in a fibrous membrane. Intramembranous bone is formed in the following manner:
a. At the site of bone formation, mesenchymal cells become aggregated.
b. Mesenchymal cells lay down bundles of collagen fibers.
c. Osteoblasts secrete a gelatinous matrix called osteoid around the collagen fibers.
d. They deposit calcium salts into the osteoid leading to conversion of osteoid into bone lamella.
e. Now the osteoblasts move away from the lamella and a new layer of osteoid is secreted which gets calcified.
g. Osteoblasts get entrapped between 2 lamellae they are called osteocytes.

Bone is a mineralized connective tissue that performs the functions of support, protection, locomotion. Bone constitutes an important reservoir of minerals.

COMPOSITION OF BONE

- Inorganic   – 65%
- Organic   – 35%
- Collagen   – 88-89%

- Noncollagen — 11-12%
- Glycoprotein — 6.5-10%
- Proteoglycans — 0.8%
- Sialoproteins — 0.35%
- Lipids — 0.4%

STRUCTURE OF BONE

- Bone consists of bone cells present in a bone matrix.
- Bone matrix or the intercellular substance is made of collagen fibers and ground substance, i.e. complex mucopolysaccharides.
- Inorangic or crystalline part of bone comprises hydroxyapatite crystals.
- Bone cells are called osteocytes and are found distributed throughout the matrix.
- Osteocytes are found occupying small spaces in the matrix called lucunae.
- Lacunae are connected to one another by a system of canals called canaliculi.
- Canaliculi open into certain canals that contains capillaries.
- Mature bone is formed in thin layers called lamellae.
- Lamellae are arranged in concentric circles called Haversian system.
- Haversian system consists of a concentric lamellae around a central canal called Haversian canal which contain capillary blood vesels.

Three distinct types of bone lamellae are found. They are:
1. *Circumferential lamellae:* They are bony lamellae that surround the entire bone, forming its outer perimeter.
2. *Concentric lamellae:* Form the bulk of the bone and form the basic metabolic unit of bone called osteon. Osteon is a cylinder of bone found oriented along the long axis of the bone.
3. *Interstitial lamellae:* They are lamellae found between adjacent concentric lamellae.

They are filters that fill the space between the concentric lamellae.

Number of canals are found in this bone. These canals are called Volkmann's canals.

Branches of blood vessels from these canal may enter smaller Haversian canals.

ALVEOLAR PROCESS

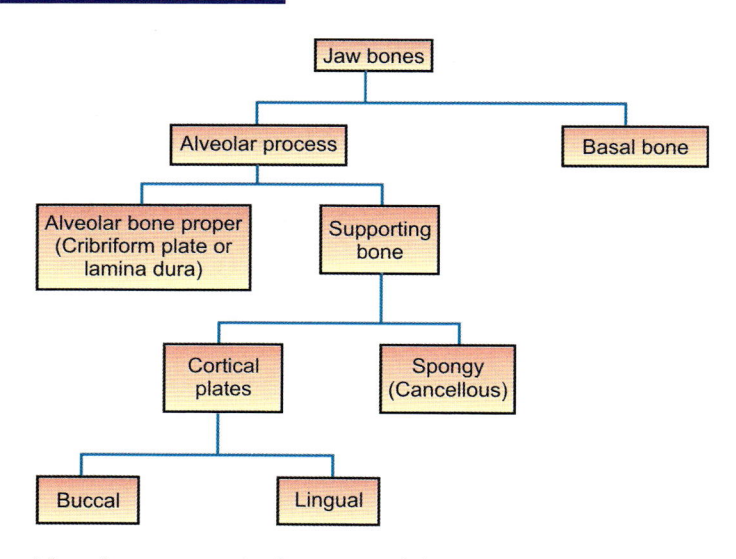

```
                    Jaw bones
                   /         \
          Alveolar process    Basal bone
           /            \
Alveolar bone proper   Supporting
(Cribriform plate or      bone
    lamina dura)        /      \
                  Cortical    Spongy
                   plates   (Cancellous)
                   /    \
               Buccal  Lingual
```

Alveolar process is that part of the jaws which support and attach the teeth. It has 2 parts:
1. *Alveolar bone proper:* Forms the socket wall and gives attachment to periodontal ligament.
2. *Supporting bone:* Consists of buccal and lingual cortical plates and the cancellous bone in between these plates and the socket walls.

CORTICAL PLATE

Cortical plate of alveolar process is continuous with cortical plate of basal bone.

These are mature lamellated bone.

Consists of dense, lamellated Haversian systems.

At the mouth of tooth sockets the surface cortical bone is continuous with the alveolar bone proper.

Thickness varies in different persons, in different arches, in different areas of the Jaws, in different aspect of the arch.

THE SPONGIOSA

Lies between the cortical plates and alveolar bone proper.

Contains marrow spaces and is continuous with the spongiosa of the body of the jaws.

Maxilla has more cancellous bone than mandible, it is more on lingual aspect than on buccal aspect, frequently absent in anterior region.

Transmits the masticatory forces from alveolar bone proper to cortical plates.

Inter-radicular and interdental septae consist entirely of spongy bone.

These septae transmit blood vessels and the radiolucent lines of these on radiographs are called Hirshfeld's canals.

Trabeculae tend to be arranged in a horizontal plane near the alveolar bone.

They are perpendicular in the inter-radicular area.

CRIBRIFORM PLATE OR THE ALVEOLAR BONE PROPER

It is the layer of compact bone which forms the bony wall of the tooth socket. It appears radiopaque in radiograph and is called Lamina dura.

It is sieve like and transmits numerous blood vessels and nerves and is called cribriform plate.

Consists of bundle and lamellated bone.

Gives attachment to Sharpey's fibers.

BONE CELLS

Osteoblasts

Connected with bone formation.

Found where new bone is forming.
Active in the formation of collagen fibrils and ground substance that constitute organic matrix.
They also take part in calcification.
Produce a homogenous intercellular substance called primary osteoid tissue.

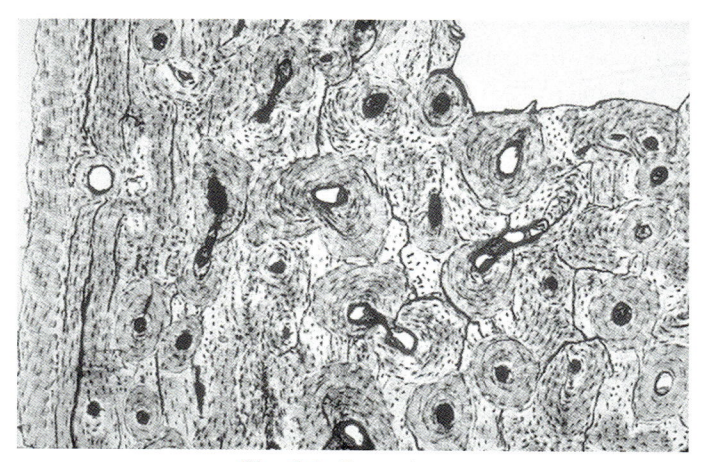

Fig. 8.1: Bone tissue
(Compact bone showing Haversian systems)

Osteocytes

Osteoblasts become entrapped in osteoid tissue during its formation and are termed osteocytes.

Occupy a space called lacuna and anastomose with each other by means of processes contained in canaliculi.

Process of osteocytes communicate with each other and with central canal of Haversian system.

Osteoclasts

Are large multinucleated connective tissue cells and are active in bone resorption.

Seen in areas undergoing bone resorption and reside in irregular scalloped surfaces of bone known as Howship's lacunae.

Osteoclasts are foreign body giant cells clearing up the debris after removal of inorganic salts.

CLINICAL CONSIDERATIONS

It is the biologic plasticity that enables the orthodontist to move teeth .

Bone resorbed on the side of pressure and apposed on the side of tension.

During healing of fracture or extraction, an embryonic type of bone is formed, which later is replaced by mature bone.

Bone resorption is common in periodontal disease.

It is universal, occurs frequently in posterior teeth, usually symmetrical, occurs in episodic spurts, is both of the horizontal and vertical type.

Once the alveolar bone is lost, it is difficult to repair or regenerate.

Oral Mucous Membrane

Chapter 9

ORAL CAVITY CONTAINS

- Teeth
- Salivary gland
- Taste buds
  It serves a variety of function.

PHYSIOLOGY OF ORAL CAVITY

- First food is tasted, masticated and mixed with saliva. Hard inedible particles are sensed and expectorated.
- Saliva secreted into the oral cavity, lubricates the food and facilitates swallowing. Enzymes in the saliva initiate digestion.
- Then food enters the digestive tract through the oral cavity.
- Body cavities are lined by mucous membranes, which are coated by serous and mucous secretion.
- Structure of oral mucous membrane varies in an apparent adaptation to function in different regions of the oral cavity.

CLASSIFICATION
(BASED ON THE FUNCTIONAL CRITERIA)

It is divided into three major types:
  i. Masticatory mucosa – Gingiva and hard palate

ii. Lining or reflecting mucosa – Lip, cheek, vestibular fornix, alveolar mucosa and soft palate
iii. Specialized mucosa – Dorsum of the tongue and taste buds.

The masticatory mucosa is bound to bone and does not stretch. It bears forces generated when food is chewed.

The lining mucosa is not equally exposed to such forces. It covers the musculature and is distensible, adapting itself to the contraction and relaxation of cheeks, lips and tongue and to movements of the mandible produced by the muscles of mastication.

The specialized mucosa (sensory mucosa) is so called because it bears the taste buds, which have a sensory function.

Oral mucous membrane is composed of:
- Epithelium
- Connective tissue.

Connective tissue component is called lamina propria. Epithelium and connective tissue form an interface that forms corrugated papillae.

Papillae of connective tissue protrude toward the epithelium carrying blood vessels and nerves.

Epithelium does not contain blood vessels. Epithelium in turn is formed into ridges that protrude towards the lamina propria.

These ridges interdigitate with the papillae and are called epithelial ridges.

At the junction there are two different structures with very similar names:
- Basal lamina
- Basement membrane.

Basal lamina is evident at the electron microscope level and is epithelial origin.

Basement membrane is evident at the light microscopy. It is found at the interface of epithelial and connective tissue with in the connective tissue.

It is a zone that is 1-4 µm wide and is cell free. This zone stains positively with the PAS method indicating that it contains "Neutral mucopolysaccharides", i.e.(Glycosaminoglycans). It also contains fine argyrophilic reticulin fibers, as well as special anchoring fibrils.

Lamina Propria

It may be described as a connective tissue of variable thickness that supports the epithelium.
It is divided into:
- Papillary
- Reticular.

Papillary portion is named for the papillae. This layer helps in increasing the area of attachment between the epithelium and the lamina propria.

The length of the connective tissue papillae vary from region to region. An increase in length of papillae is seen in areas where additional, mechanical adhesion is required between the epithelium and the lamina propria, e.g. masticatory mucosa.

In areas where not much masticatory load falls the papillary layer is smaller while the reticular layer is larger.

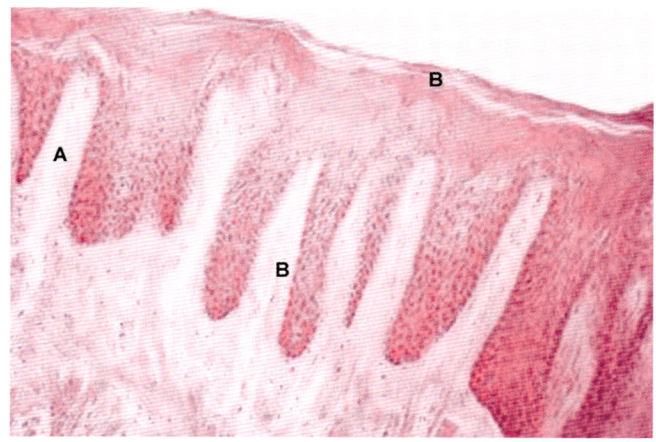

Fig. 9.1: Oral mucous membrane (A) Connective tissue papillae (B) Keratinized layer (stratum corneum) of stratified squamous epithelium

Capillary loops are seen extending into the papillary layer of lamina propria. As the epithelium is a avascular layer, its needs are met by the rich vascular subepithelial plexus of the underlying papillary layer of lamina propria.

The lamina propria is attached to the periosteum of the alveolar bone or may overlay the submucosa.

Submucosa

The submucosa is a connective tissue of variable thickness that serves primarily as attachment for the lamina propria to the underlying bone or muscle.

The submucosa contains glands, adipose tissue and also the vascular and neural components. The submucosa contains a deep plexus of large blood vessels which branch into smaller vessels and reach the subepithelial plexus. The blood vessels are accompanied by lymphatic channels. Lymph nodes can be occasionaly found in the roof of the tongue and between the glossopalatine and pharyngopalatine arches.

Numerous myelinated nerves are seen in the submucosa. They loose their myelin sheath before they terminate.

Masticatory Mucosa

The masticatory mucosa covers the areas of the oral cavity that are exposed to compressive and shear forces and to abrasion during mastication. The hard palate and gingiva are covered by masticatory mucosa.

Hard Palate

It is covered by masticatory mucosa. The epithelium is well keratinized and appear pink. Underlying the epithelial layer is the lamina propria which differs in thickness from region to region of the hard palate.

The hard palate can be subdivided into several zones based on the nature of the underlying submucosa.

They are:
- Median palatine raphe

Oral Embryology and Histology

- Rugae
- Gingival region
- Anterolateral fatty region
- Posterolateral glandular region.

Mid palatine raphe does not contain submucosa. The dense lamina propria directly attaches to the underlying bone.

The gingival region of the hard palate is the peripheral zone of the palate immediately adjacent to the palatal gingiva.

In this zone too the submucosa is absent.

Rugae appears in the anterior regions of the palate on either side of the mid line. They are seen as irregular, asymmetric ridges of mucous membrane. Rugae do not cross the mid line and can be easily seen and palpated.

Histologically the rugae are folds of epithelium with dense connective tissue extensions. These bands are called traction bands and they make the rugae immovable.

In the anterolateral regions of the hard palate the submucosa is rich in fatty adipose tissue.

In the posterolateral areas of the palate the submucosa is filled with glandular tissue. The glandular zone extends upto the soft palate. Glands are usually of mucous type.

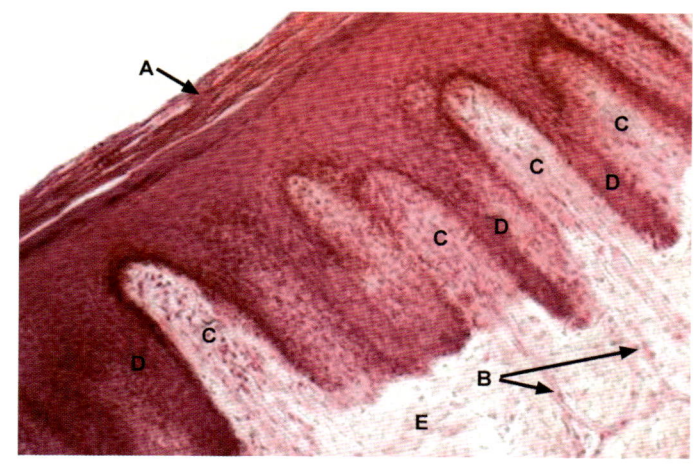

Fig. 9.2: Histology of hard palate (A) Stratum corneum (B) Capillary (C) Connective tissue papilla (D) Rete peg (E) Lamina propria

The incisive papilla is a dense elevation seen in the anterior region of the hard palate behind the maxillary central incisors. It contains dense connective tissue and ducts of varying length.

These ducts are the vestigial nasopalatine duct that are lined by pseudostratified and stratified columnar epithelium. Minor mucous salivary glands may occasionally open into these ducts.

Gingiva

It is that part of mucosa which surrounds the tooth and covers the alveolous.

The gingiva is divided into 2 regions depending on the firmness with which it is attached to the underlying tissue.

About 1-15 mm of coronal part of the gingiva is loosely attached to the tooth and is called free gingiva.

The potential space between tooth and free gingiva is called gingival sulcus or gingival crevice. Viewed from facial or lingual aspects the margins of free gingiva, appears as a wavy line and is known as marginal gingiva. The free gingiva in the interproximal area is known as papillary gingiva or interproximal gingiva.

The gingiva apical to the free gingiva is firmly attached to the underlying structure via gingival fibers of periodontal ligament called attached gingiva.

The junction of free and attached gingiva produces a scalloped depressed line known as free gingival groove, which runs parallel to the margin of gingiva.

The surface of the attached gingiva has a stippled or a pitted appearance.

Microscopic Features of the Gingiva

Broadly speaking the gingiva is made up of epithelium and connective tissue.

It is studied under – Outer oral epithelium
– Sulcular epithelium
– Junctional epithelium

Outer Oral Epithelium

This comprised of the crest and outer surface of the free gingiva and the surface of the attached gingiva.

Epithelium consists of following layer

1. Stratum basale – Cuboidal to columnar stem cells. Useful in replacing lost cells.
2. Stratum spinosum – Large polyhedral cells which are connected by spine like process.
3. Stratum corneum – Most superficial keratinized layer, cells are flat, lacking nucleus.

The various cell of the gingiva are attached to one another by: (1) Desmosomes (2) Zona occludens (3) Gap junctions.

Sulcular Epithelium

It lines the gingival sulcus and extends from the coronal area of the junctional epithelium to the free margin of gingiva.

It is nonkeratinized, but can undergo keratinization on prolonged antibiotic therapy.

Junctional Epithelium

As the tooth erupts, the reduced enamel epithelium over the tip of the erupting teeth degenerates there by creating the space for eruption.

In this place reduced enamel epithelium combines with oral epithelium and called Junctional epithelium.

It consists of stratified squamous nonkeratinized epithelium of 3-4 cell thickness and length of 0.25-1.35 mm.

Junctional epithelium has three zones:
1. Apial zone
2. Middle zone
3. Coronal zone.

Oral Mucous Membrane

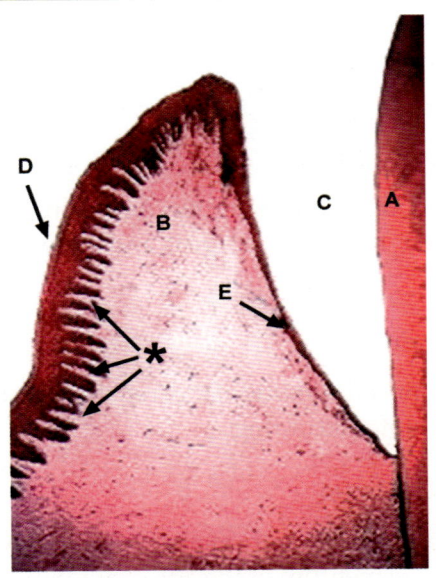

Fig. 9.3: Histology of gingiva *Connective tissue papillae (A) Dentin (B) Gingiva (C) Enamel space (D) Keratinized stratified squamous epithelium (E) Sulcular epithelium

Gingival Sulcus

It is formed during eruption of tooth into the oral cavity. It is a shallow 'V' shaped space or groove that encircles newly erupted teeth and extends from coronal to the junctional epithelium being bound inside by the tooth and outside by the sulcular epithelium.

Gingival or Sulcular Fluid

This is a fluid that seeps from the gingival connective tissue. It has antimicrobial properties and helps to clean the sulcus.

It also contains plasma proteins which help in increasing adhesion of the epithelial attachments.

Connective Tissue of Gingiva

It is also called lamina propria and lies below the epithelium.

Connective tissue contains numerous bundles of collagen which helps in holding the gingiva firmly.
They are:

A. *Gingivo Dental Group*

These are fibers originate from the cementum and project in a fan-like manner towards the crest and outer surface of free gingiva.

B. *Circular Group*

Found in the connective tissue of the free and interdental gingiva encircling the tooth like a ring.

C. *Trans-septal Group*

Located interproximally and extend between the cementum of one tooth to the cementum of the adjacent tooth above the inter dental bone.

Connective tissue also contains fibroblasts capable of regenerating and destroying collagen fibers.

Even in normal gingiva, the connective tissue contains plasma cells, lymphocytes and neutrophills. This is due to infiltration of antigens from the sulcus to the connective tissue.

Lining Mucosa

It covers most parts of the oral cavity. It is made up of thick non-keratinized epithelium and a thin zone of lamina propria.

Lip and Cheek

Mucous membrane is nonkeratinized stratified squamous epithelium. Lamina propria consists of dense connective tissue.

Papillae are short and regular. Minor salivary glands are also seen. Larger glands lie in the buccinator muscle of cheek.

Isolated sebaceous glands are seen as whitish spot and known as Fordyce's granules.

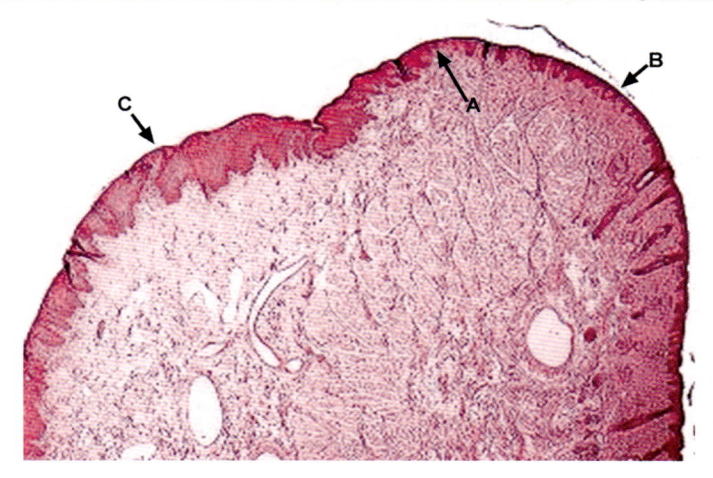

Fig. 9.4: Histology of lip (A) Mucocutaneous junction (B) Skin of the lip (C) labial mucosa

Vestibule and Alveolar Mucosa

Epithelium is nonkeratinized stratified squamous. Mucosa is loosely attached to the underlying structure and periosteum.

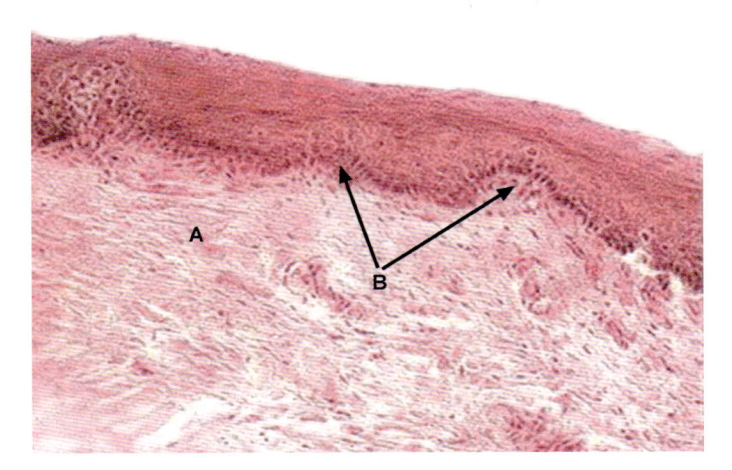

Fig. 9.5: Histology of alveolar mucosa (A) Lamina propria (B) Connective tissue papillae

Alveolar mucosa, is separated from gingiva by a scalloped line called mucogingival junctions.

Ventral Surface of Tongue and Floor of Oral Cavity

The epithelium is nonkeratinized. Connective tissue papillae of lamina propria are very short. Submucosa contains fat and salivary glands.

Mucosa of ventral surface of tongue is thin. Papillae are numerous and short. The submucosa is indistinguishable from lamina propria. The mucosa is bound tightly to muscles of tongue.

Dorsal Surface of Tongue

Tongue is divided grossly into:
- Anterior 2/3rd and
- Posterior 1/3rd.

It is divided by a 'V' shaped line, the sulcus terminalis. Anterior part is covered by a keratinized stratified squamous epithelium forming different papillae.

Papillae are Four Types

- Filiform
- Fungiform
- Foliate
- Vallate.

Filiform Papillae

About 2.5 mm and are conical in shape. The epithelial covering of these papillae are thick.

It also consists of loose connective tissue core covered by a keratinized stratified squamous epithelium.

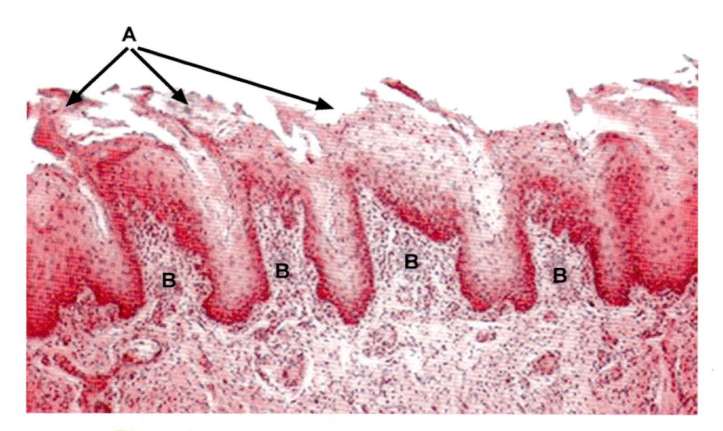

Fig. 9.6 : Filiform papillae (A) Keratinized layer (B) Connective tissue core

Fungiform Papillae

They are short, flat shaped and dome shaped. They are about 2 mm long and 1 mm wide.

Number is much smaller than that of filiform papillae.

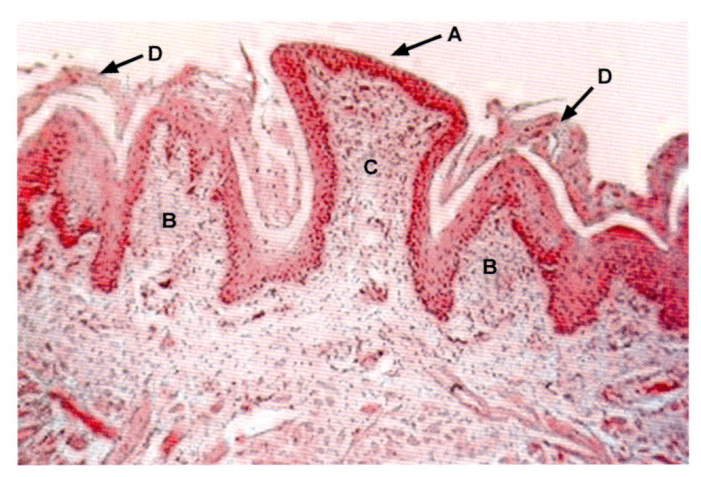

Fig. 9.7: Fungiform papillae (A) Fungiform papilla (B) Filiform papillae (C) Connective tissue core (D) Keratinized layer on filiform tip

Foliate Papillae

Seen parallel to lateral mucosal folds near the posterior part of the body of the tongue.

They are well-developed at birth but become rudimentary during adult life.

4-8 in number and bear taste buds.

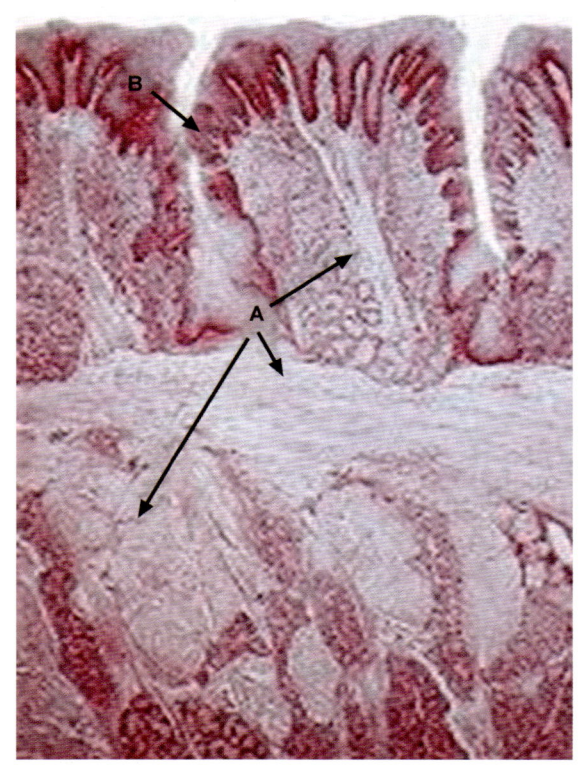

Fig. 9.8: Foliate papillae
(A) Skeletal muscle fibers (B) Taste buds

Vallate (Circumvallate) Papillae

These are largest of the papillae. About 1 mm height and 2.5 mm wide.

They are mushroom-shaped and situated just anterior to the sulcus terminalis.

10-12 in number Angle of 'V' shows a depression called foramen caecum.

The papillae as well as crypt are lined by stratified squamous epithelium.

Papillae consists of collagen fibers. Taste buds number about 250 in each papillae.

The albuminous glands of von Ebner empties their secretion in the crypt.

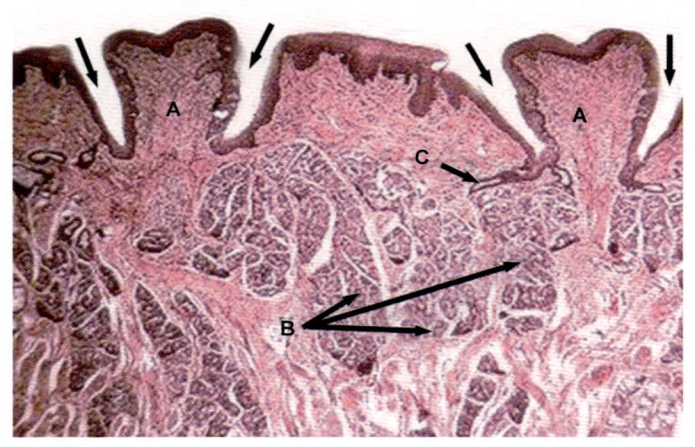

Fig. 9.9: Circumvallate papillae (A) Circumvallate papilla (B) Glands of von Ebner (C) Duct of glands of von Ebner

Taste Buds

These are seen in the papillae, mucosa of soft palate and Pharynx. They are barrel-shaped structures surrounded by stratified squamous epithelium.

It consists of 2 types of cells, the taste cells and supporting cells. The taste buds are intraepithelial, the cells lying perpendicular to the basement membrane.

There are 4-20 taste cells/bud. They are thin columnar cells, also known as gustatory or neuroepithelial cells.

Posterior 1/3rd of the tongue shows a number of irregular elevations called lingual follicles. They are lymph nodules. The lingual follicles together called lingual tonsils.

Taste Determination

- Circumvallate	Papillae	Bitter taste
- Foliate	Papillae	Sour taste
- Fungiform	Papillae	Salty taste at the lateral sides of tongue
- Filiform	Papillae	Sweet taste at the top of the tongue.

Salivary Glands

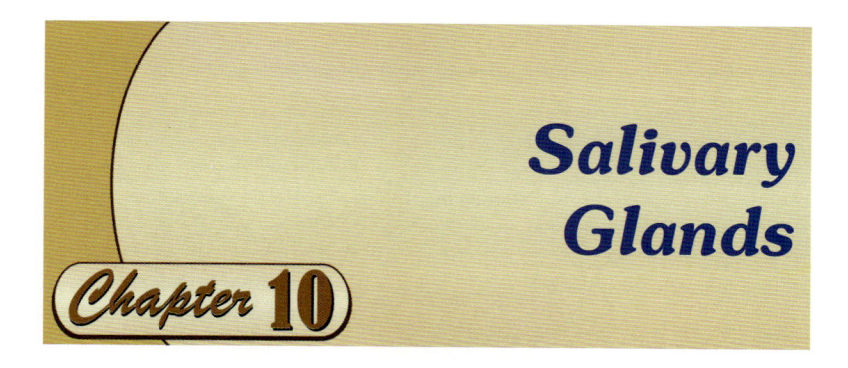

Chapter 10

ANATOMY OF SALIVARY GLANDS

A. *Parotid gland* is the largest
   - Situated in front of the ear and behind the ramus of the mandible.
   - Weight, 14-28 gm. Intimately associated with peripheral branches of facial nerve.
   - Duct opens into the oral cavity in a papillae opposite to the maxillary second molar.
B. *Submandibular gland* weighs around 10-15 gm.
   - Situated in the posterior part of the floor of the mouth.
   - Duct opens by the way of a small orifice lateral to the lingual frenum.
C. *Sublingual gland* is almond shaped.
   - Weight, 2 gm, situated in the floor of the mouth between the side of the tongue and the teeth.
   - Series of small ducts are seen.
D. All minor salivary glands except serous gland of von Ebner are found below the sulci of circumvallate papillae and in the foliate papillae of tongue.

Major Salivary Glands

   i. *Parotid gland:* This is enclosed in a capsule with its superficial portion lying in front of the external ear and its deeper part filling the retromandibular fossa.

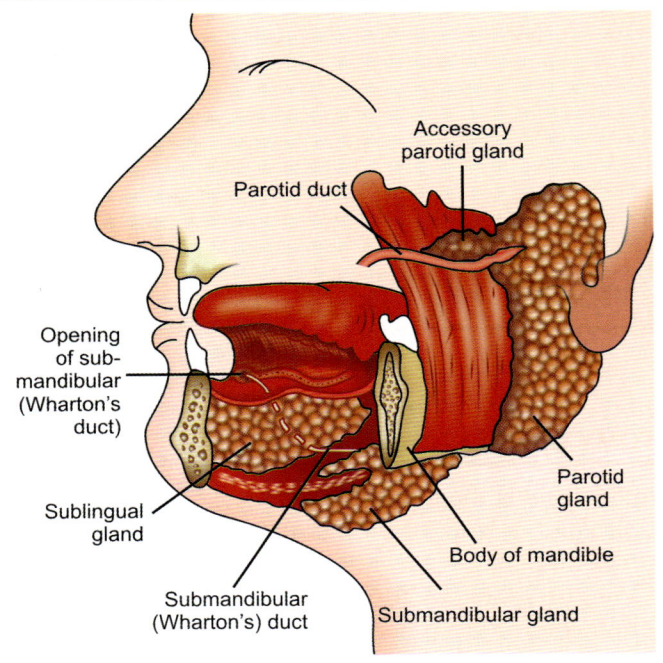

Fig. 10.1: Anatomy of salivary glands

Excretory duct—*Stenson's duct*

Purely serous in adults but a few mucous secretory units may be found in the infants.

ii. *Submandibular gland:* It is also enveloped by a well-defined capsule located in the submandibular triangle behind and below the free border of the mylohyoid muscle with a small extension lying above the mylohyoid.

Excretory duct—Wharton's duct (opens at caruncula subligualis).

Mixed type (Predominantly serous).

The intercalated duct tends to be somewhat shorter than parotid but striated duct is usually longer.

iii. *Sublingual gland:* Lies between the floor of the mouth and the mylohyoid muscle.

Excretory duct—Bartholin's duct

Mixed type (Predominantly mucous)

Minor Salivary Glands

- These glands produce mucoprotein rich secretion except serous glands of von Ebner.
- Play a role in the formation of acquired pellicle.
- There is occurrence of focal accumulation of lymphocytes around their ductal walls which are thought to have role in the immune surveillance of the mouth.

a. Labial and buccal glands – Mixed type consisting of mucous tubules with serous demilunes.

b. Glossopalatine glands – Purely mucous.

c. Palatine glands – Purely mucous. Found on the posterolateral region of the soft palate and uvula.

d. Lingual glands – Anterior part called glands of Blandin and Nuhn located near the apex of the tongue. Chiefly mucous and duct opens on to the dorsal surface of tongue.

– Posterior part called gland of von Ebner's, located between the muscle fibers of the tongue below the vallate papillae. Duct opens into the trough of vallate papillae. purely serous.

Development of Salivary Glands

The primordia of the parotid glands appear during 4th week of fetal life, whereas primordia of submandibular and sublingual appear around 6th-8th week of fetal life.

Minor salivary glands begin their development during 3rd month.

Development begins with a downgrowth of epithelium from the lining of the stomodeum.

This forms a solid cord of cells that grows into the underlying mesenchyme and branches to form multiple epithelial strands with bulbous terminus which leads to form secretory endpieces.

Later the centers of the solid strands are followed by degeneration of the cell so that by 6 months an intact ductal system has formed.

Secretrion commences at around birth.

Histology and Structure of the Salivary Glands

In a fully developed gland the histological appearance resembles to a branch of grapes divided into lobules by connective tissue septa.

Connective tissue septa carry main blood vessels, nerves and large interlobular ducts.

Interlobular duct drains into a single excretory duct which discharges saliva into the mouth.

Lobules of epithelial component is arranged into closely packed secretory units.

These units actively secrete the saliva and consist of a group of cells arranged around a central lumen.

Two types of secretory cells are seen:
  i. Serous
  ii. Mucous.

Serous Cells

Characterized by rounded compact endpieces called acini, which contains numerous basophilic secretory granules on routine staining.

These are specialized form of cells characterized by pyramidal in shape, with its apex situated towards the central lumen and broad base resting on a thin basal lamina.

Nucleus is spherical and is situated in the basal 1/3rd of the cell.

Salivary Glands 109

Occasionally binucleated cells are observed.

These are specialized for the synthesis, storage and secretion of proteins.

It has large amount of rough endoplasmic reticulum arranged in parallel stacks packed basally and laterally to the nucleus.

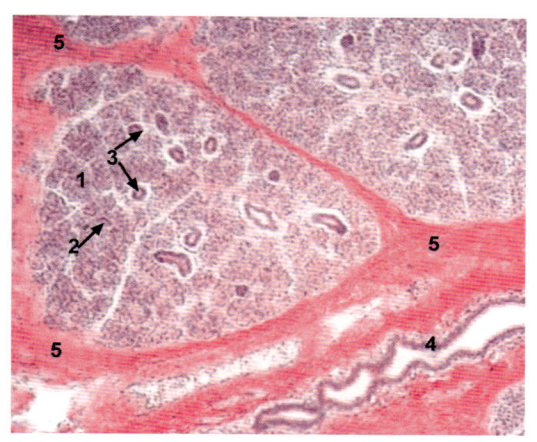

Fig. 10.2A: Histology of serous cells under low magnification (Parotid gland)

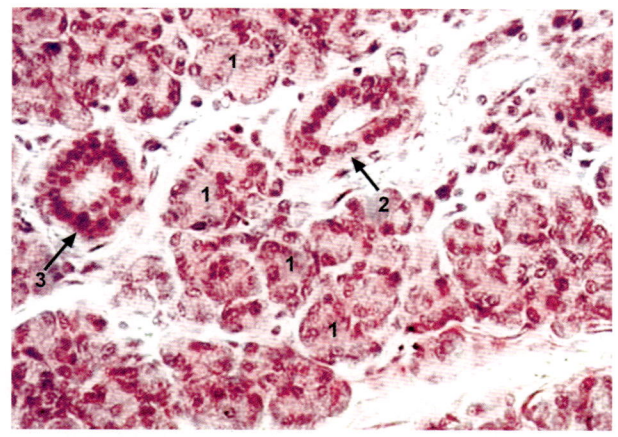

Fig. 10.2B: Histology of serous cells under high magnification (Parotid gland) (1) Serous secretory units (2) Striated excretory duct (3) Interlobular excretory duct

Also has a prominent Golgi complex situated apically and laterally to the nucleus.

Most prominent feature of serous cell is the accumulation of secretory granules called **zymogen granules** in the apical cytoplasm.

These secretory granules are discharged by a process called *Exocytosis*.

Mechanism of Action of Exocytosis

Fusion of the granular membrane with plasma membrane at the lumen or intercellular canaliculus occurs.
↓
Followed by opening of the fused portion
↓
Granular membrane becomes continuous with plasma membrane
↓
Granule content is excreted without loss of cytoplasm.

COMPOUND EXOCYTOSIS

This is a process of rapid secretion which occurs during stimulation by various pharmacologic agents.

A second granule may fuse with the membrane of a previously discharged granule.

Apical part of the cytoplasm is filled with zymogen granules and appears eosinophilic in a H&E stain.

Identification Point of Serous Cell

- Composed of round acini with small lumen.
- Nucleus is spherical and present at basal 1/3rd.
- Apical cytoplasm stain eosinophilic because of secretory granules.

Salivary Glands 111

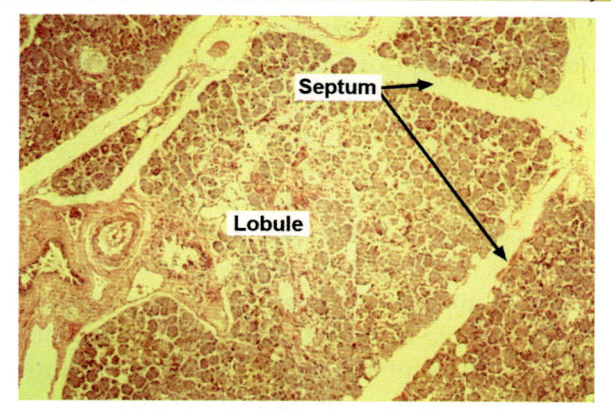

Fig. 10.3A: Histology of mixed salivary gland (Submandibular gland) under low magnification

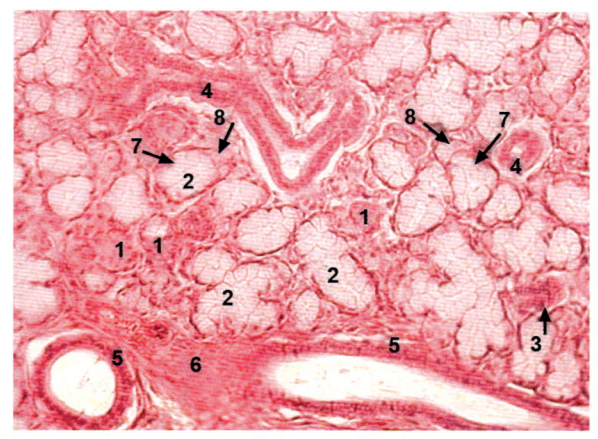

Fig. 10.3B: Histology of mixed salivary gland (Submandibular gland) under high magnification (1) Serous secretory unit (2) Mixed secretory unit (3) Intercalated excretory duct (4) Striated excretory duct (5) Interlobular excretory duct (6) Interlobular connective tissue septa (7) Mucous part of mixed secretory unit (8) Serous part (serous demilune) of mixed secretory unit

Mucous Cells

Characterized by plump polygonal cells with a clear, mucous filled cytoplasm. They usually form short tubular structures referred as *Tubuloacini*.

Many of the mucous endpieces are surrounded by serous cells to form serous caps or DEMILUNES, which drain into the same lumen.

These are the cells having numerous secretory units called mucous acini, which is a collection of mucous cells.

columnar in shape with nucleus flattened and pressed against the basement membrane.

Cytoplasm is restricted to basal region apical portion of the cell is filled with mucous secretory droplets and appears empty in H and E stain, due to higher carbohydrate content.

Cells are ovoid or tubular in shape with large lumen.

The secretory products of most mucous cells differ from those of serous cells in 2 important aspects.
   i. Mucous have little or no enzymatic activity and probably serve mainly for lubrication and protection of the oral tissue.
   ii. The ratio of carbohydrate to protein is greater and larger amounts of sialic acid and occasionally sulfated sugar residues are present.

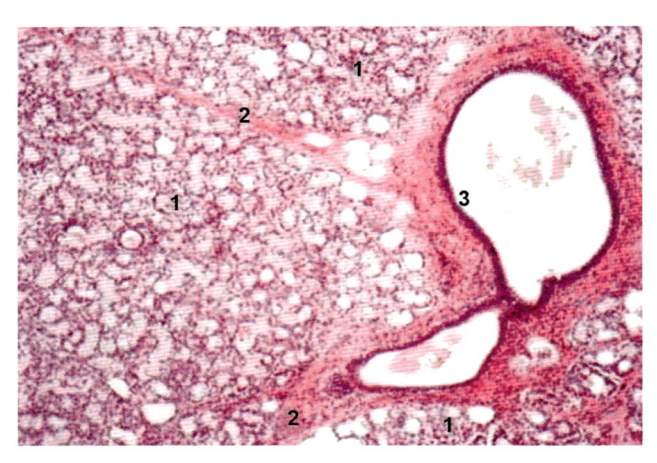

Fig. 10.4A: Histology of mucous salivary gland under low magnification (1) Lobules of the gland (2) Interlobular connective tissue septa (3) Interlobular excretory duct

Salivary Glands

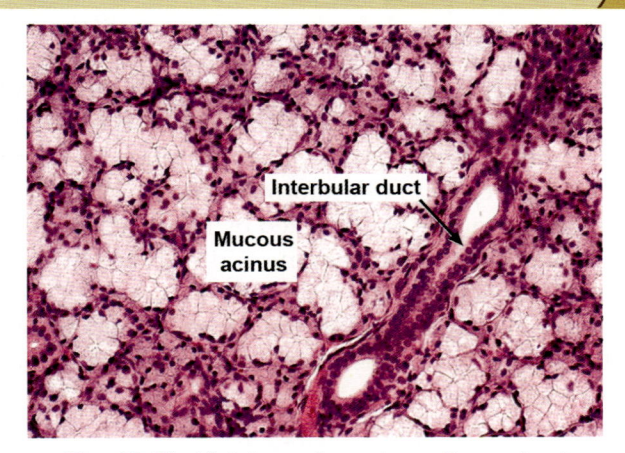

Fig. 10.4B: Histology of mucous salivary gland under high magnification

Identification of Mucous Glands
- Composed of tubular acini with large lumen
- Nucleus of cells is flat and pressed
- Apical cytoplasm appears empty
- Ultastructurally mucous cells contain more prominent Golgi complex which reflect the cell in increased carbohydrate metabolism and its secretory material is stored in droplets.

Applied Aspect
These myoepithelial cells play an important role in formation of pleomorphic adenoma and myoepithelioma, where the characteristic myxoid or mucous stroma is of myoepithelial origin.

STRUCTURE AND FUNCTION OF SALIVARY GLAND CELLS

The terminal secretory units are composed of serous, mucous and myoepithelial cells.

These cells are arranged into acini or secretory tubules.

Myoepithelial Cells

These are special type of cells, contractile in nature and have some feature of smooth muscles. Its function is to support the secretory units and may also facilitate secretion by contracting and causing the ejection of preformed saliva.

Secretory endpieces are invested by myoepithelial cells that lie within the basement membrane and embrace the acini and intercalated ducts with long branching processes.

These are closely related to the secretory and intercalated duct cells, lying between basal lamina and basement membrane of the parenchymal cells.

Usually one myoepithelial cell per secretory endpiece is found but 2-3 may be seen.

Morphology varies according to its location.
A. If associated with intercalated ducts then, there will be spindle shaped cell and have fewer processes.
B. If associated with secretory endpiece, then it shows an image of octopus sitting on a rock.

Desmosomal atttachments are present between the myoepithelial cells and underlying secretory cells.

Arrangement of Cells in the Terminal Secretory Units

Terminal secretory unit differs from gland to gland.
  i. In a serous gland the cells are clustered in a roughly spherical fashion around a central lumen forming an acinus.
     - At the apical part the lumen is sealed off from the lateral intercellular spaces by junctional complexes.
     - Three junctional complexes are seen
       A. Tight junction—Zonula occludens.
       B. Intermediate junction—Zonula adherens.
       C. One or more desmosomes—Maculae adherens.

This prevents leakage of the luminal contents into the intercellular spaces.

Salivary Glands 115

During secretion the junctions become permeable to macromolecules and organic substances.

ii. In a mucous gland, the arrangement of secretory cells is similiar but rather than a spherical acinus a tubular secretory endpiece is seen.

Ducts of Salivary Gland

Three types of ducts are seen, namely:
- Intercalated duct
- Striated duct
- Main excretory duct

$$\text{Terminal endpiece} \\ \downarrow \\ \text{Intercalated duct} \\ \downarrow \\ \text{Striated duct} \\ \downarrow \\ \text{Terminal excretory duct}$$

Intercalated Duct

These are of smaller diameter and are lined by a single layer of low cuboid cells with relatively empty appearing cytoplasm and centrally placed nucleus.

Difficult to identify because they are compressed between secretory units.

Rough endoplasmic reticulum are seen basally and Golgi complex apically.

Striated Duct

Lined by a layer of tall columnar cells which have centrally placed nuclei and eosinophilic cytoplasm.

Prominent striation at the basal ends are seen.

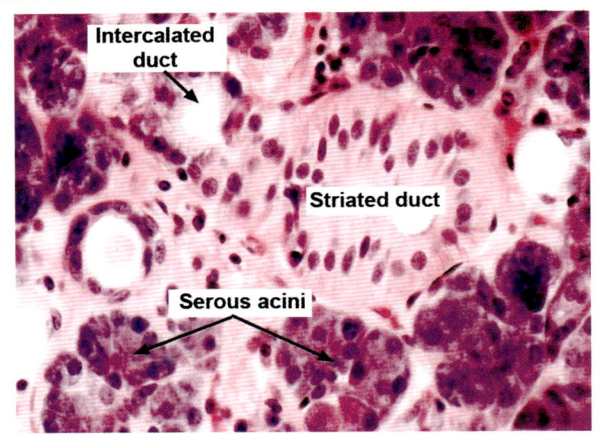

Fig. 10.5: Diagram showing intercalated and striated ducts

Terminal Excretory Duct

Histology varies as they pass from the striated ducts to the oral cavity.

Near the striated duct it is lined by a pseudostratified epithelium consisting of tall columnar cells.

As the duct approaches the oral cavity, epithelium gradually changes to a true stratified epithelium.

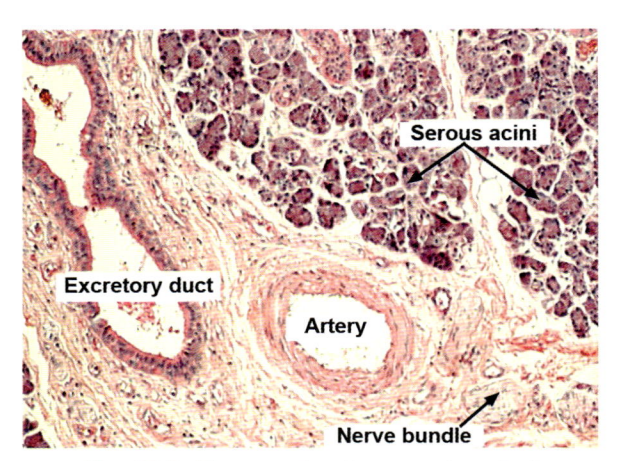

Fig. 10.6: Diagram showing excretory duct

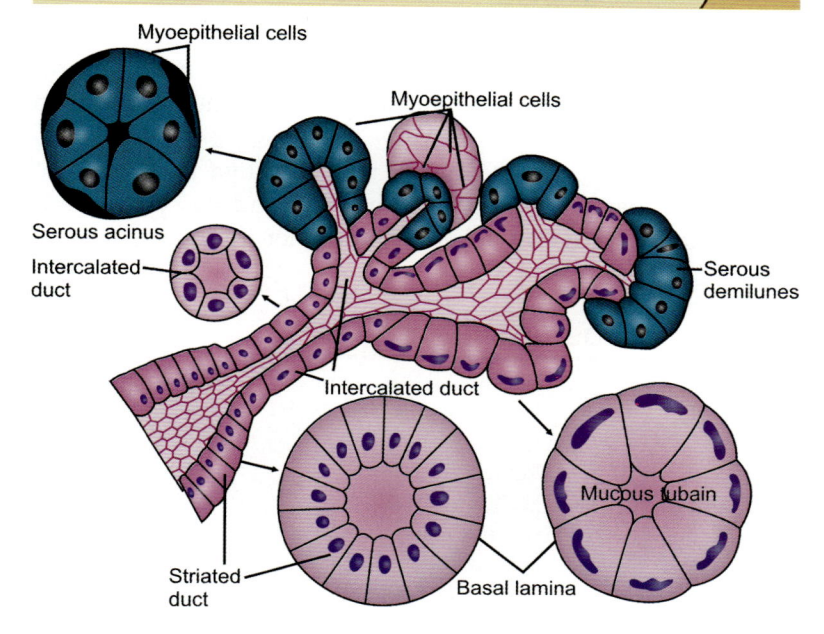

Fig. 10.7: Diagram representing ductal system of salivary gland

Functions of Salivary Ducts

1. Convey the primary saliva secreted by the terminal secretory units to the oral cavity.
2. Actively modify the primary saliva by reabsorption of electrolytes and secretion of protiens.
3. Antibacterial protiens like lysozyme and lactoferrin are secreted from the intercalated duct.
4. Striated duct contains kallikrein, an enzyme found in saliva and synthesize secretory glycoproteins.

Connective Tissue Elements

It contains fibroblasts, macrophages, mastcells, occasional leukocytes, fat cells and plasma cells.

These cells are embedded in proteoglycans and glycoprotein like ground substances.

Blood vessels are also seen.

The vesicles are believed to contain the chemical neurotransmitters norepinephrine and acetylcholine and release them by process of exocytosis.

In general, a copious flow of watery saliva is secreted in response to parasympathetic stimulation and by sympathetic stimulation it releases thicker saliva higher in organic content and less in quantity.

SALIVA COMPOSITION AND FUNCTION

i. Protection	- Lubrication - Water proofing - Lavage - Pellicle formation	- Glycoprotein - Water
ii. Buffering	- Maintains pH unsuitable for colonization - Neutralizes acid	- Phosphates and bicarbonates
iii. Digestion	- Bolus formation - Neutralizes esophageal contents and digests starch	- Phosphates and bicarbonates - Amylase
iv. Taste	- Solution of molecules - Taste bud growth and maturation	- Water - Gustin
v. Antimicrobial	- Barrier effect - Antibody - Hostile environment	- Glycoprotein - IgA, IgG, IgM - Lysozyme and lactoferrin
vi. Tooth integrity	- Enamel maturation and repair	- Calcium, phosphate and fluoride

The pH of whole saliva varies from 6.7-7.4 whereas parotid saliva varies from 6.0-7.8.

Clinical Considerations

With an exception of a portion of the anterior part of the hard palate, salivary glands are seen everywhere in the oral cavity.

Salivary Glands | 119

Sometime the glands occur in an area just posterior to the 3rd molar teeth.

In maxilla salivary glands may be seen in the nasopalatine canal.

Common Disease Seen

- Inflammatory
- Viral
- Bacterial
- Allergic
- Benign and malignant tumors
- Autoimmune diseases like-Sjögren syndrome
- Genetic diseases – Cystic fibrosis
- Obstructive diseases – Mucocele
- Systemic and metabolic diseases.
- Salivary glands especially major may become enlarged during starvation, protein deficiency, alcoholism, pregnancy, diabetes mellitus and liver disease
- Xerostomia – Absence or reduction of salivary flow.

Maxillary Sinus

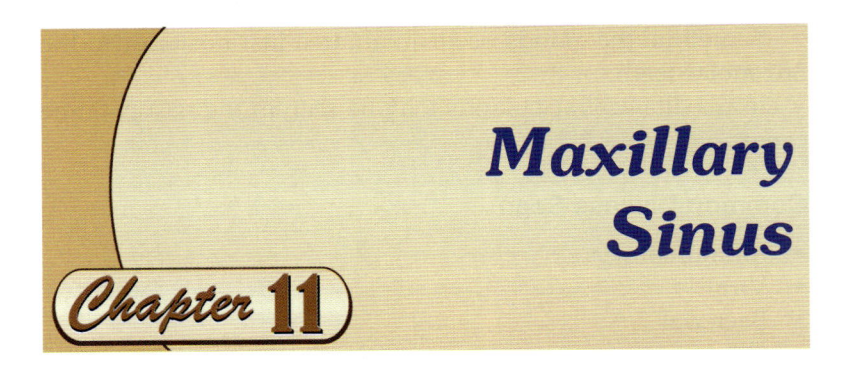

Chapter 11

INTRODUCTION

It is a pneumatic space lodged inside the maxilla that communicates with the environment by way of middle nasal meatus and nasal vestibule.

Otherwise known 'Antrum of highmore'.

Because Highmore was the first to describe the maxillary sinus morphology in detail and about the idea of pneumatization by the sinuses.

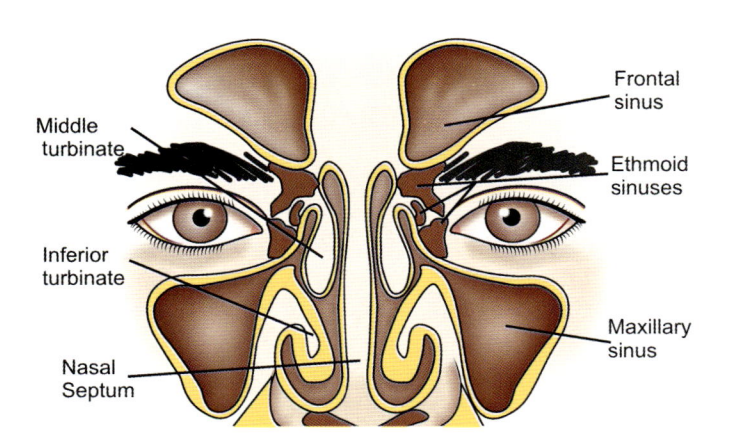

Fig. 11.1: Paranasal sinuses

STRUCTURE AND VARIATION

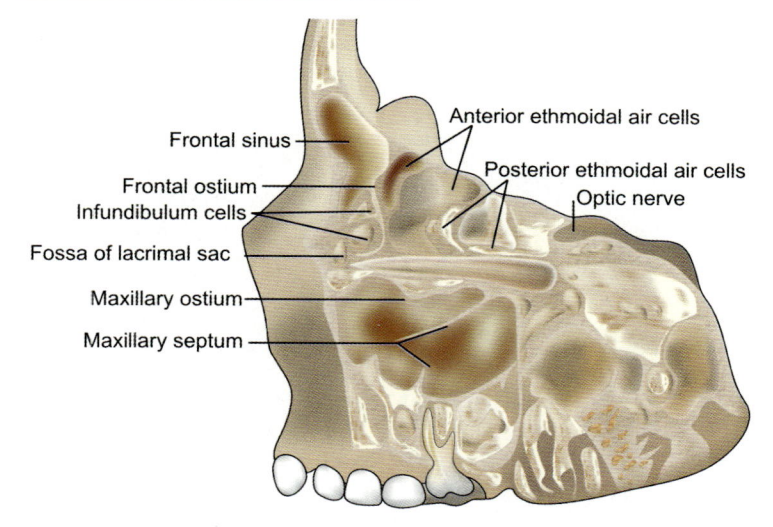

Fig. 11.2: Anatomic location of maxillary sinus

Maxillary sinus is subject to a great extent of variation in size, shape and mode of developmental pattern.

Sinus is described as a four sided-pyramid;
- Base – Faces medially to nasal cavity.
- Apex – is pointed laterally towards the body of the zygomatic bone.

Four sides are related to the surface of the maxilla in the following manner:
a. Anterior : To the facial surface of the body of maxilla.
b. Posterior : To the infratemporal surface.
c. Superior : To the orbital surface .
d. Inferior : To the alveolar and zygomatic process.

Four sides of sinus are usually distant from one another medially, but converge laterally to meet at an obtuse angle.

Base of the sinus is the thinnest of all walls and it presents a perforation, the ostium at the level of middle nasal meatus.

In some individuals in addition to the main ostium, two (or) more accessory ostia connect the sinus with the middle nasal meatus.

The latter development of maxillary sinus most often pneumatizes the floor of the sinus adjacent to the roots of the first molar and less often to roots of 2nd premolar, 1st premolar and 2nd molar in that order of frequency.

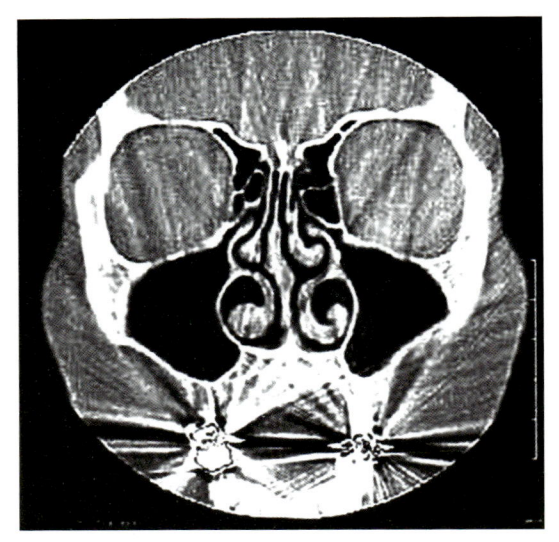

Fig. 11.3: Radiographic view of maxillary sinus (Paranasal view)

Microscopic Features

Three distinct layers surrounding the space of the maxillary sinus is seen:
a. Epithelial layer
b. Basal lamina
c. Subepithelial layer, including the periosteum.

Epithelium is of a pseudostratified, ciliated and columnar type—derived from the olfactory epithelium of the middle nasal meatus.

Cellular type usually seen are ciliated columnar cells and in addition to these basal cells, nonciliated columnar cells, and mucous-producing secretory cells (Goblet cells) are also seen.

Ciliated cells consist of a nucleus and electron lucent cytoplasm and numerous mitochondria and enzyme containing organelles.

Cilia

- Cilia are composed of 9+1 pairs of microtubules.
- It provides the motile apparatus for the sinus.
- By the way of ciliary beating, the mucous blanket lining the epithelium, moves into the nasal cavity from the sinus.

Goblet Cells

Goblet cells exhibit the characteristic features of secretory cells.

In its basal segment it consists of a nucleus, rough and smooth endoplasmic reticulum and Golgi apparatus.

Zymogen granules in Golgi apparatus transport the mucopolysacchrides to the cellular apex and finally releases it by exocytosis to the epithelial surface, along with a mixed secretory product.

[(i.e.) a serous secretion consisting primarily of water with little amounts of nonspecific lipids, proteins, carbohydrates].

This serous secretion is produced by subepithelial glands present in subepithelial layer, which, enters the lumen of sinus by excretory ducts which first pierce the basal lamina.

FUNCTIONS OF MAXILLARY SINUS

If air is arrested in the sinus, it soon charges to body temperature, thus protecting internal structures, such as the brain, particularly, from exposure to cold air.

Contributes to the—
- Resonance of the voice.
- Lightening of skull weight.
- Enhances the faciocranial resistance against mechanical shock.
- Production of the bactericidal lysozyme to the nasal cavity.

CLINICAL CONSIDERATIONS

Developmental Anomalies

Agenesis (Complete absence)
 Aplasia and hypoplasia (altered development and under development).
 In association with cleft palate, high palate, septal deformity, mandibulofacial dysostosis.

Larger Sinuses

Larger sinuses in case of pituitary gigantism.
 Congenital infections by spirochaeta in congenital syphilis – small sinuses

Oroantral Fistula

Upperfirst molar closest to floor of maxillary sinus, hence surgical manipulation of the tooth break through the partitioning bony lamina thus oroantral fistula.
- 2.19% –   by 1st molars
- 2.01% –   by 2nd molars.

If left untreated the lumen of fistula epithelialize and permanent communication of oral cavity with maxillary space occurs.

Other Causes for Oroantral Fistula

Radicular cyst, granuloma (or) abscess in relation to molar or premolar.
 Hypercementosis of root apices and subsequent extraction may lead to perforation. Hence, radiograph is necessary to determine the relationship between any such premolar (or) molar with the floor of maxillary sinus prior to surgical intervention.
 Chronic infections of mucoperiosteal layer of sinus might involve superior alveolar nerves, if they are closely related to the sinus and cause neuralgia. Diagnosis in this instance must be based on careful inspection of all upper teeth.
 Malignant lesions such as adenocarcinoma, squamous cell carcinoma osteosarcoma may produce pain, loosening, supraeruption or bleeding in their gingival tissue.

Temporo-mandibular Joint

Chapter 12

It is formed by the articulation between the articular tubercle and the anterior part of mandibular fossa of temporal bone above and condylar head of the mandible below.

The articular disk is interposed between articular surfaces of the two bones.

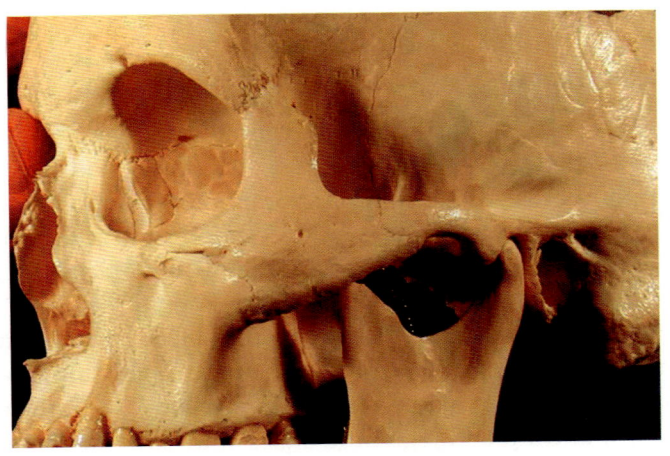

Fig. 12.1: Temporomandibular joint

ARTICULAR DISK

- It is oval, fibrous plate that fuses at its anterior margin with the fibrous capsule.

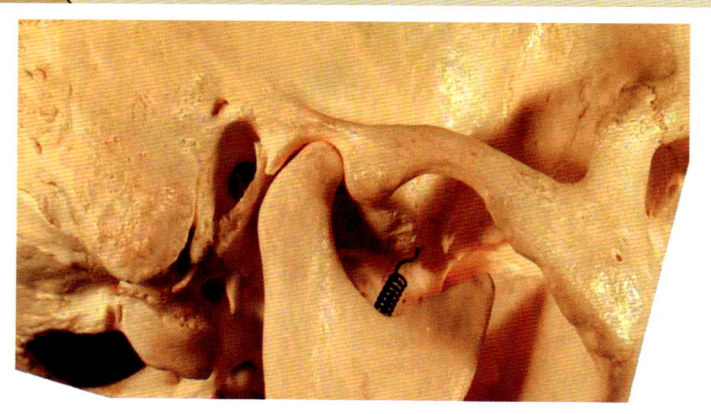

Fig. 12.2: Diagram showing condyle, coronoid process, glenoid fossa, infratemporal region and zygomatic arch

- Posterior border is connected to the capsule by loose connective tissue which allows its anterior movement.
- Medial and lateral borders (corners) are attached to poles of the condyle.

Articular Space

Articular space is divided into two compartments:
a. Lower: Between condyle and the disk (Condylodiscal)
b. Upper: Between disk and temporal bone (Temporodiscal)
   - Disk is biconcave in sagittal section with a thin intermediate zone, a thick posterior band and a thick anterior band.

Latter is continuous with a loose—fibroblastic portion called bilaminar zone, which is highly vascular and highly innervated.

Superior stratum of bilaminar zone attaches to the posterior wall of mandibular or glenoid fossa and squamotympanic suture.

Articular capsule is a fibrous sac:
   Attaches anteriorly—to articular tubercle
   Posteriorly—to lips of squamotympanic fissure.
- Articular capsule is strengthened laterally by temporomandibular ligament.

- Inner aspect of capsule is lined by synovial membrane.
- It lines the capsule in each of the two cavities and doesn't extend over disk surfaces, articular tubercle, or condyle.

DEVELOPMENT OF THE JOINT

- At 10 weeks: Components of the future joint show the first indication in mesenchyme between condylar cartilage of the mandible and developing temporal bone.
- At 12 weeks: Two slit-like joint cavities and an intervening disk appear in this region.
- The mesenchyme around the joint begins to form the fibrous joint capsule.

HISTOLOGICAL FEATURES

Bony Structures

1. *Condyle of mandible*
   - Composed of cancellous bone and covered by a thin layer of compact bone.
   - Trabeculae are grouped in such a way, that they are radiating from the neck of the mandible and reach cortex at right angles.

   Marrow spaces are large and decrease in size on ageing by thickening of trabeculae.
   - Red marrow in the condyle is of myeloid (or) cellular type.
   - Period of growth shows a hyaline cartilage beneath the fibrous capsule of condyle. This cartilage grows by apposition from the deepest layers of the covering connective tissue. This at same time is replaced by bone in its deep surface.

2. *Roof of the mandibular fossa:* Consists of a thin, compact layer of bone.

3. *Articular tubercle:* Composed of spongy bone covered with a thin layer of compact bone. Rarely islands of hyaline cartilage are found.

ARTICULAR FIBROUS COVERING

- Condyle and articular tubercle is covered by a fibrous tissue containing varying numbers of chondrocytes.
- Fibrous covering is of fairly even thickness superficial layer consists of strong, collagenous fibers.
- Chondrocytes may be present and they increase in number with age.
- Chondrocytes are recognized by their:
  1. Thin capsule.
  2. Staining heavily with basic dyes.
- Deepest layer of fibrocartilage – Rich in chondroid cells as long as hyaline cartilage is present in the condyle.

(In this zone, appositional growth of hyaline cartilage of condyle takes place).

- Fibrous layer covering the articulating surface of the temporal bone is thin in articular fossa and thickens rapidly on the posterior slope of articular tubercle.
- In this region the fibrous tissue is seen to be of two different layers with a transitional zone between.

Inner layer: Fiber bundles run at right angles to the bone surface.

Outer layer: Fibers run parallel to the bone surface.
- Chondrocytes are found.
- Deepest layer shows thin zone of calcification.
- There is no continuous cellular lining on free surface of fibrocartilage. Only isolated fibroblasts with long, flat cytoplasmic processes are seen.

Articular Disk

Younger individuals → Composed of dense fibrous tissue.
- Interlacing fibers are straight and tightly packed.
- Elastic fibers are in small number. Fibroblasts are elongated with cytoplasmic processes (Flat and wiglike).

With Advancing Age

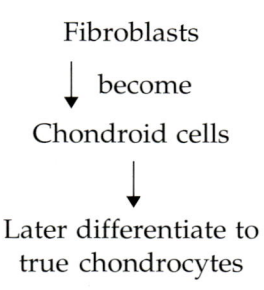

Fibroblasts
↓ become
Chondroid cells
↓
Later differentiate to true chondrocytes

- Differentiation of fibroblasts lead to development of chondroid cells, true cartilage cells, hyaline ground substances
  Presence of chondrocytes – Increases resistance and resilience of fibrous tissue.

Fibrous tissue covering the articular eminence and mandibular condyle, as well as large central area of the disk, is devoid of blood vessles, nerves, and has limited reparative ability.

ARTICULAR CAPSULE

- It consists of an outer fibrous layer that is strengthened on lateral surface to form the temporomandibular ligament.
- Lined by synovial membrane, which folds with synovial villi.
- Synovial villi projects into joint spaces.
- The synovial membrane consists of – internal cells. These don't form continuous lining instead show gaps between cells, and subintimal connective tissue, rich in blood capillaries.

It is of three types:
a. A – Rich in Golgi complex (Macrophage-like).
b. B – Rich in rough endoplasmic reticulum (Fibroblast-like).
c. A and B (Cellular morphology between types A and B).
   - A small amount of clear, straw-colored, viscous fluid is seen is articular spaces.
   - It acts as lubricant, nutrient fluid for avascular tissues covering condyle, articular tubercle and for the disk.

- It is elaborated by diffusion from rich capillary network of synovial membrane.
- Augmented by mucin secreted by synovial cells.

INNERVATION AND BLOOD SUPPLY

- Sensations from joint structures are proprioceptive in nature.
- Nerve supply   –   Auriculotemporal nerve
                    –   Masseteric nerve
                    (From the mandibular branch of trigeminal nerve)
- Primitive source   –   Superficial temporal artery
  of blood supply   –   Maxillary artery

CLINICAL CONSIDERATIONS

1. Thinness of bone in articular fossa – Responsible for fractures if mandibular head is driven into the fossa by a heavy blow.
   - In such cases dura mater and brain have been reported to result in injuries.
   - Change in direction of a force or a stress may cause structural changes.
   - Degeneration of fibrous covering of articulating surfaces and of the disk. Hence, compensation and partial repair is accomplished by development of hyaline cartilage on condylar surface and in the disk.
   - Severe trauma to articular bone is destroyed, cartilage and new bone develop in marrow spaces and at the periphery of the condyle. Then function of joint is severely impaired.
2. Myofacial pain dysfunction syndrome (Dysfunction of the temporomandibular joint).

Features

1. Masticatory muscle tenderness (Mostly lateral pterygoid and then temporalis, medial pterygoid and masseter in order).

2. Limited opening of the mandible (less than 37 mm).
3. Joint sounds.

Causes

- Masticatory muscle spasm.
- Stress related.

Treatment

- Slinting.
- Occlusal grinding/reconstruction.
- Invasive therapy.

Dislocation

- Usually bilateral and displacement is anterior.

Example

While yawning, the head of mandible may slip forward into the infratemporal fossa causing articular dislocation of the joint.

Tooth Eruption

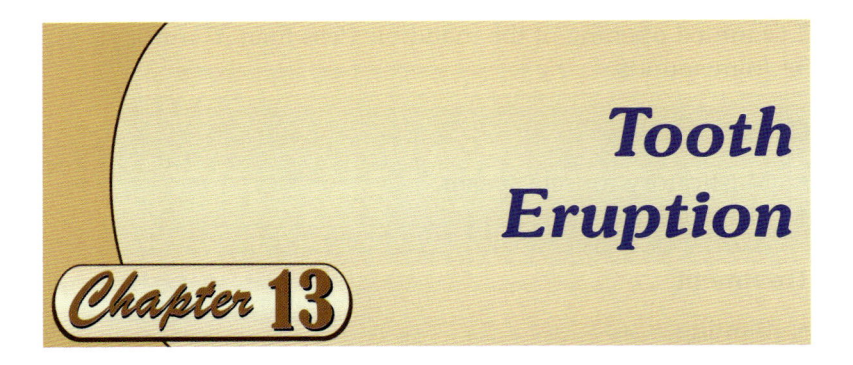

Chapter 13

Teeth develop within jaws.

For teeth to become functional, movement is required to reach the occlusal plane.

Movement of teeth is divided as:

PRE-ERUPTIVE MOVEMENT

Movement made by deciduous and permanent tooth germs before eruption.

ERUPTIVE TOOTH MOVEMENT

Axial/occlusal movement of the tooth from its developmental position within the jaws to its functional position in the occlusal plane.

POSTERUPTIVE MOVEMENT

i. Maintain the position of erupted tooth in occlusion while the jaws grow.
ii. Compensate for occlusal proximal wear.

A. Pre-eruptive Movement

Aim

Movements required to place the teeth within the jaw in a position for eruptive tooth movement.

Involves

1. Bodily movement of tooth germs.
2. Growth of tooth germs.
3. Relative change in the position of permanent and deciduous tooth germs.

Example

1. *Deciduous tooth germs:* Initially small space between them. With tooth germs growth, crowding occurs – relieved by growth of jaws – second deciduous molars move backwards, move forward. They also move outwards, downward or upward as the jaws increase in length, width and height.
2. Successional permanent teeth develop on lingual aspect of deciduous predecessor in the same bony crypt – they shift from here, occupy their own bony crypt lingual to root of predecessors.

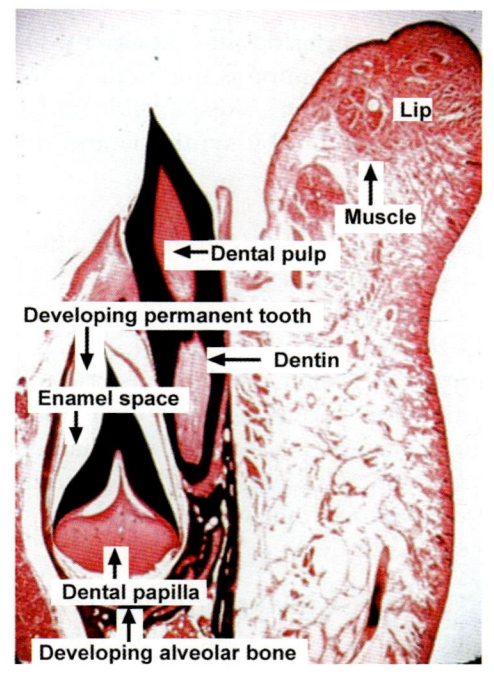

Fig. 13.1: Pre-eruptive tooth movement

3. Permanent molar teeth germs without predecessor, e.g. upper molar initially develop with occlusal surfaces facing distally – after maxillary growth – comes to position.

Mandibular molar – initially axis is tilted mesially after jaw growth – becomes vertical.

Histology of Pre-eruptive Phase

Deposition and resorption of bone, e.g. bodily movement in a mesial direction—resorption on mesial surface of crypt wall and deposition on distal surface due to osteoclastic and osteoblastic activity.

B. Eruptive Movement

Movement from position within the jaws to occlusal/functional position.

Histology of Eruptive Phase

1. Formation of roots, periodontal ligament, tooth eruption begins when root formation is initiated.
2. Structural changes in PDL—Responsible for tooth eruption.
   i. Remodelling of PDL by synthesis and degradation of collagen.
   ii. *Fibroblasts have:*
      a. Intermediate filaments with contractile properties.
      b. Cell—cell contacts.
      c. Close relationship between fibroblasts and ligament collagen bundles.
      d. *Fibronexus:* Term used to describe morphologic relationship between intracellular filaments, transmembrane proteins, extracellular filament fibronectin.
      e. Fibronectin: Sticky glycoprotein, permits adhesion of fibroblasts to extracellular components. All these help in tooth eruption.

Changes in Tissues Overlying Erupting Tooth

Initially, bone surrounds the tooth germs, but does not cover completely.

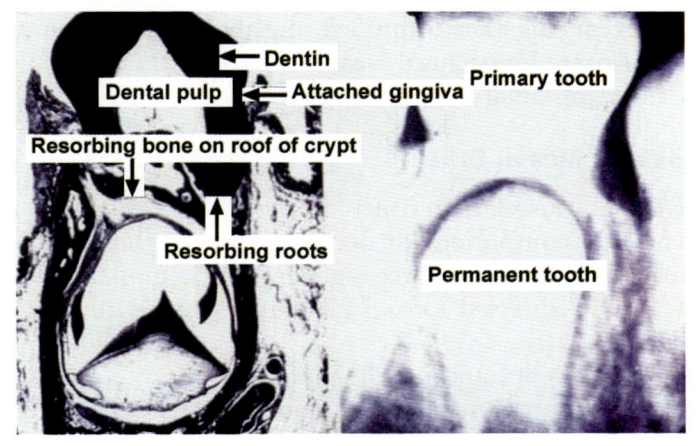

Fig. 13.2: Eruptive tooth movement

As deciduous predecessors erupt, permanent teeth shift apically, enclosed by bone except for a canal – called gubernacular canal, which contains connective tissue, remnants of dental lamina called gubernacular cord.

Suggested that gubernacular canal is rapidly widened by local osteoclastic activity delineating the eruptive pathway for the tooth.

C. Posteruptive Phase

Tooth makes movements to:
1. Compensate for growth of jaws.
2. Compensate wear (occlusal, interproximal wear).
   Readjustment of tooth socket position.

Histology of Posteruptive Phase

Formation of new bone at alveolar crest and on socket floor – to compensate for increasing height of jaws.

This is however not responsible for tooth movement.

Compensation of Occlusal Wear

- Cementum deposition at apices but it occurs only after tooth has moved.

- Forces causing tooth eruption bring about axial movement – compensate for occlusal wear.
- Mesial/proximal drift.

Causes for Mesial Drift

(Forces that cause mesial drift)
1. Anterior component of occlusal force: When teeth are brought into contact, force is generated in a mesial direction. Anteriorly directed force is generated which will move the teeth mesially.
2. Contraction of transeptal ligament.
3. Soft tissue pressures—cheeks and tongue.

Histological Features

Compensation for proximal wear is seen as selective deposition and resorption of bone on the socket walls.

Under Electron Microscope

Remodelling of collagen in periodontal and transeptal ligaments.

THEORIES OF TOOTH ERUPTION

a. Root Formation/Root Growth Theory

Was thought to be the cause for eruption.

Against this Theory

1. Rootless teeth erupt.
2. Some teeth erupt a greater distance than the length of their roots.
3. Teeth have been found to erupt after root completion or after Hertwig's root sheath and periapical tissue have been removed surgically.
4. If root growth has to be responsible for eruption, the apical growth of the root has to be translated into an occlusal movement it requires the presence of a fixed base.

However, bone at the base resorbs if pressure is applied.
Investigators thought that a cushion—Hammock ligament straddling the base of the socket from one bony wall to the other act as a fixed base.
But histologically, no such structure was found.

b. Vascular Pressure—Hydrostatic Pressure Theory

Teeth move synchronously with arterial pulse.
Increase in pressure either within or around the base of tooth during tooth eruption (i.e. vasculature is responsible for eruption).

Against this Theory

Surgical excision of a growing root and associated tissues eliminates periapical vasculature – however eruption is not impeded.

Bony Remodelling Theory

Selective deposition and resorption of bone in crypt wall – eruption.

EXPERIMENTS

If a developing tooth is removed without disturbing its dental follicle – an eruption pathway forms within bone.
If dental follicle is removed, no eruptive pathway forms.
Therefore, dental follicle is necessary for bony remodeling.

Dental Follicle

1. Provides vascular route for osteoclasts (derived from monocytes) to reach the crypt wall.
2. Reduced enamel epithelium – Epidermal growth factor + Transforming growth factor (Cytokines) – stimulate follicular cells to express colony stimulating factor – recruit osteoclasts to follicle – resorption of bone.

Periodontal Ligament Traction Theory

Force for eruptive movement is in PDL (Periodontal ligament).

Experimental Evidence

1. Lack of vitamin C: ↓ collagen during eruption stopped/slowed.
2. Injecting agents interfering with cross-linking of collagen → eruption stopped/slowed.
   Periodontal ligament important → for eruption.

Fibroblasts in periodontal ligament have:
1. Contractile properties
2. Cell—cell contact
3. Fibronexuses bywhich contractile force is transmitted to collagen bundles. Contraction of fibroblasts → force transmitted to adjacent fibroblasts → summation of contractile forces → through fibronexuses → force transmitted to collagen bundles → remodelling → eruptive movement.

CLINICAL CONSIDERATIONS

Premature Eruption

- Neonatal teeth/Natal teeth → Teeth present at birth.
- Premature loss of deciduous teeth → early eruption of permanent successors.
- Delayed eruption → causes
  i. Congenital
  ii. Systemic
     – Nutritional
     – Genetic
     – Endocrine.

Local Factors

1. Early loss of deciduous teeth → drifting of adjacent teeth → prevents eruptive pathway.

2. Increased density of fibrous tissue arround tooth → delays eruption.
3. Impacted teeth, embedded teeth, Ankylosed teeth.
4. Orthodontic movement.

Plasticity of the tooth supporting tissues → helps in orthodontic treatment pressure side → resorption, leading to remodeling of collagen → tooth movement.

Shedding of Deciduous Teeth
Chapter 14

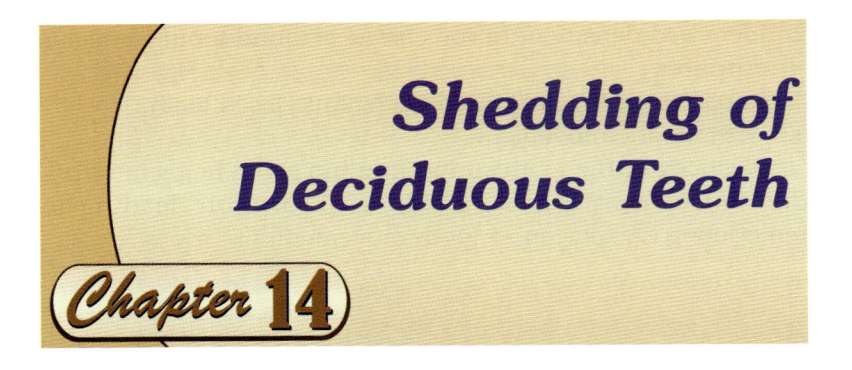

The physiologic process resulting in the elimination of the deciduous dentition is called shedding or exfoliation

Resorption of roots and periodontal ligament causes shedding (Fig. 14.1).

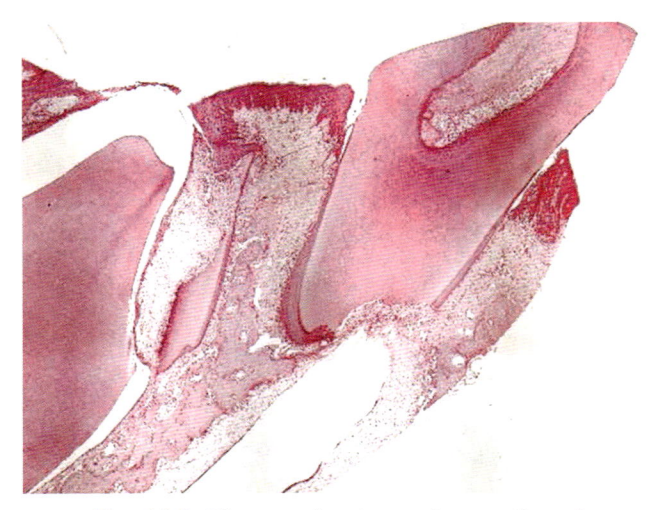

Fig. 14.1: Diagram showing root resorption of deciduous tooth

The pressure generated by the developing permanent tooth germ governs the pattern of deciduous tooth resorption.

Examples

- Permanent incisor and canine tooth germs are initially on the lingual surface of the roots of corresponding deciduous teeth.

↓

- Therefore, pressure exerted by the permanent tooth germs causes resorption of the root of the corresponding deciduous teeth on the lingual surface.

↓

- Later, permanent tooth germs shift apical to their deciduous predecessors.

↓

- Erupt in place of their deciduous predecessor.
- Resorption of roots of deciduous molar begins on their inner surface as permanent bicuspid tooth germs is found between the roots.

↓

- Later, permanent bicuspid tooth germ shifts to an apical position.

Odontoclasts

- Cells identical to osteoclasts
- Resorb dental hard tissues
- Multinucleated cells
- Vacuolated cytoplasm
- "Ruffled border" present on the cell surface adjacent to the resorbing hard tissue
- Increased acid phosphatase
- Mineral crystallites are found with in the deep invaginations of the ruffled border.

Origin

Monocyte

Location

On the surface of roots in relation to the advancing permanent tooth.

Root canals and pulp chambers of resorbing teeth.

Mechanisms of Resorption and Shedding

Pressure from the erupting successional tooth is one factor causing resorption of deciduous tooth.

Forces of mastication applied to the deciduous tooth can initiate resorption.

Events in Resorption of Hard Tissue

Removal of mineral followed by extracellular dissolution of organic matrix (mainly collagen).

Pattern of Resorption

Single rooted teeth—shed before root resorption is complete. Molars—roots are completely resorbed and the crown is partially resorbed prior to exfoliation.

CLINICAL IMPLICATIONS

Deciduous Teeth Remnants

Cementum, dentin of deciduous teeth may remain embedded in the jaw, especially in lower second premolar regions.

Cause

Parts of deciduous teeth may not be in the path of erupting permanent teeth → escape resorption → get embedded in jaw.

Retained Deciduous

Most commonly—Maxillary lateral incisors.

Shedding of Deciduous Teeth

Causes

1. Absence of permanent successors.
2. Impacted permanent successors, e.g. deciduous and permanent canine.
3. Ankylosed permanent successors.

Submerged Deciduous Teeth

Trauma to dental follicle or periodontal ligament
↓
Teeth eruption ceases
↓
Tooth gets ankylosed to bone

(i.e. there is no intervening periodontal ligament and the tooth is attached directly to bone).

Adjacent teeth erupt normally and there is increased height of the alveolar bone → therefore the ankylosed tooth appears submerged.

Deciduous II molar—Most common "submerged tooth".

Section 2

Oral Physiology

Age Changes in Dental Tissues and Jaws

Chapter 15

AGE CHANGES IN THE MANDIBLE

In Infants and Children

At Birth

a. *Mental foramen:* Opens below the sockets for the two deciduous molar teeth near the lower border.
b. *Mandibular canal:* Runs near the lower border of mandible.
c. *Angle* is obtuse (140 degrees or more).
d. *Coronoid:* Process is large and projects upwards above the level of the condyle.

In Adults

a. *Mental foramen:* Opens midway between the upper and lower border of mandible.
b. *Mandibular canal:* Runs parallel to myolohyoid line.
c. *Angle* reduces to about 110 or 120 degrees.

In Old Age

a. Teeth fall out and height of body reduced.
b. *Mental foramen and mandibular canal* are close to the alveolar border.
c. *Angle:* Becomes obtuse (140 degrees).

148 Oral Physiology

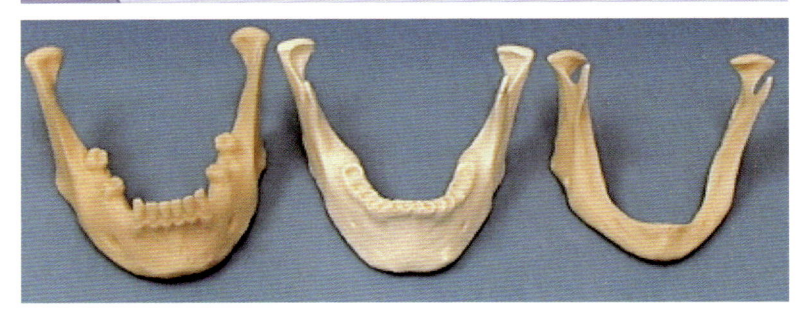

Fig. 15.1: Age changes

AGE CHANGES IN ENAMEL

Enamel is a non-vital tissue and is incapable of replacement.
1. *Most apparent age change:* Attrition or wear of the occlusal surfaces and proximal contact points as a result of mastication. Vertical dimension of crown–shortens, proximal contour–flattens.

OTHER CHANGES

Color – Teeth Darken

Cause

- Addition of organic material from the environment.
- Progressive thinning of enamel → leads to deepening of dentin color.

Permeability

- Enamel becomes less permeable with age.

Nature of Surface Layer

- Localized increases of certain elements such as nitrogen and fluorine
- Perikymata disappears
- Decreased incidence of caries.

AGE CHANGES IN DENTIN

Dentin is a Vital Tissue
1. Secondary dentin is laid down, dentin becomes thicker.
2. *Formation of sclerotic dentin (or) translucent dentin* caused by calcification of dentinal tubules → leads to increase in brittleness and decrease in permeability (Fig. 15.2).

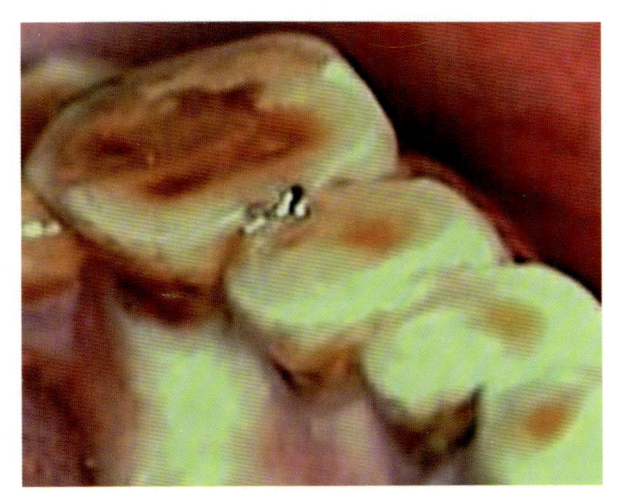

Fig. 15.2: Attrition

3. *Occurrence of dead tracts:* Dentinal tubules are emptied by either *complete retraction* of the odontoblast process from the tubule *on death* of odontoblast.
4. Dentin is exposed to oral cavity due to wearing of enamel (Fig. 15.3).

AGE CHANGES IN PULP
1. Root canal is present as a thin channel due to continued dentin deposition.
2. Cell changes – cells are characterized by decrease in size and number of cytoplasmic organelles. Number of odontoblast reduces.

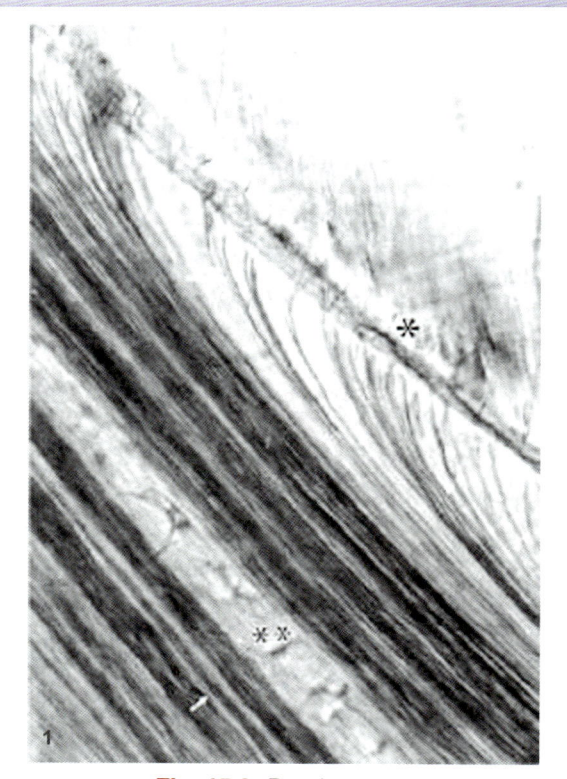

Fig. 15.3: Dead tract

3. Increase in collagen fibers
4. Reduction in the vascular supply to the pulp and calcification is seen. These calcified masses are known as pulp stones or Dentils.
5. Pulp stones are classified, according to their structure as
   i. True denticles
   ii. False denticles
   iii. Diffuse calcifications

Pulp stones may also be classified according to their location.
- Free denticles (entirely surrounded by pulp tissue)

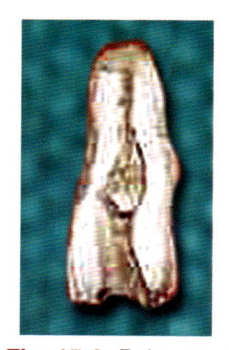

Fig. 15.4: Pulp stone

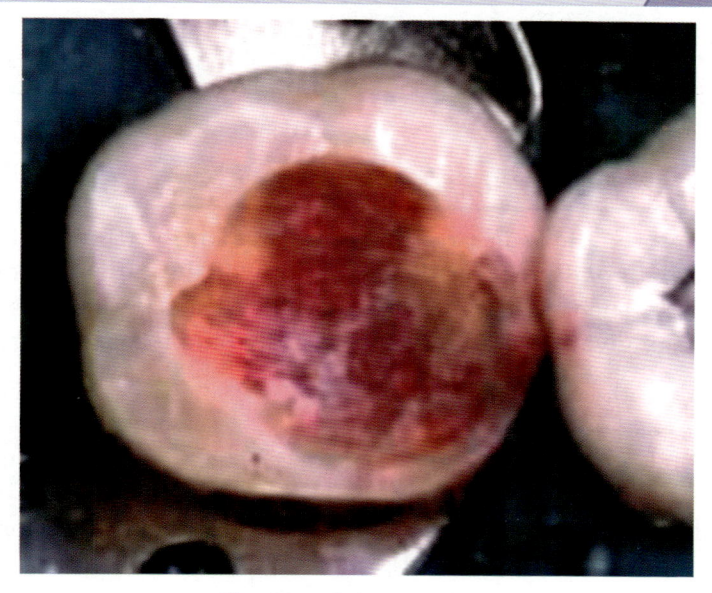

Fig. 15.5: Sclerotic dentin

- Attached denticles (partly fused with the dentin)
- Embedded denticles (entirely surrounded by dentin)
6. This loss of sensitivity.

AGE CHANGES IN PERIODONTAL LIGAMENT

Reconstruction and reorientation of the periodontal ligament to compensate for the mesial drift of teeth and increased length of root due to cementum deposition.

AGE CHANGES IN CEMENTUM

1. Cementum thickens with age due to depositional of new cementum. Non-functioning teeth—cementum may be thicker.
2. Permeability decreases.

AGE CHANGES IN ALVEOLUS

As aging occurs, alveolar bone is resorbed and height of face is reduced.

AGE CHANGES IN DENTOGINGIVAL JUNCTION

With age, there is progressive apical migration of the dentogingival junction. Exacerbations of the inflammatory focus, by such factors as poor oral hygiene, leads to gingivitis → dentogingival junction migrates apically onto the cementum.

AGE CHANGES IN ORAL MUCOSA

1. Oral mucosa has a smoother, dryer surface than in youth which is atrophic or friable.
2. Dorsum of the tongue shows reduction in number of filliform papillae and consequent prominence of foliate papillae.
3. Vascular changes quite prominent.
4. Sebaceous glands (Fordyce's spots) increase with age and the minor salivary glands show marked atrophy with fibrous replacement → lead the xerostomia.

AGE CHANGES IN SALIVARY GLANDS

1. Fatty degenerative changes, fibrosis and progressive accumulation of lymphocytes in the salivary glands.

AGE CHANGES IN TM JOINT AND MAXILLARY SINUS

1. The articular eminence flattens out.
2. Capsular ligament is lengthened due to the stress created by the loss of teeth.
3. Headache and ear symptoms occur because of the degeneration of the articular surface and articular disk.
4. The floor of maxillary sinus comes close to oral cavity with a thin bone intervening.

Effects of Hormones on the Oral Structures

Chapter 16

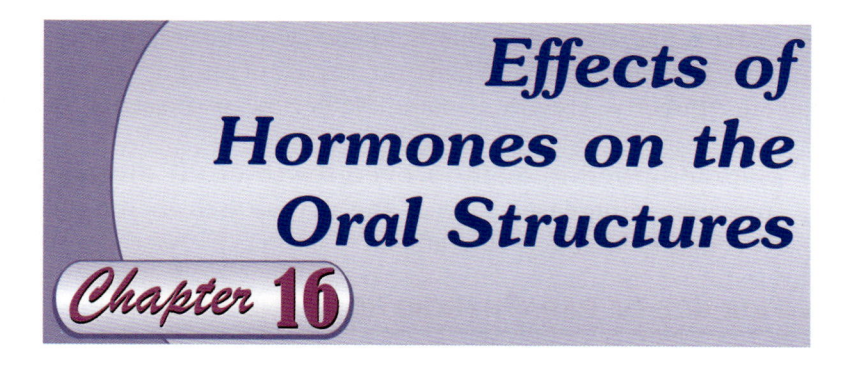

EFFECTS OF HORMONES ON THE ORAL STRUCTURES

The Thyroid Hormone

Hypothyroidism from birth → retarded growth of the skeleton → results in small dental arch.
- The size of the crown is little affected
- Eruption retarded
- Dental delay is approximately 1/3rd that of skeletal delay
- Shedding of deciduous teeth is delayed
- Growth of roots are slower than normal
- Pulp canals are unusually wide
- Mandible poorly developed → open bite and a receding chin.

EFFECTS OF GROWTH HORMONE

Growth hormone is one of the hormones secreted by the anterior pituitary.

Pituitary dwarfism causes a delay in the eruption and shedding of the teeth.
- Dental delay is approximately half that of skeletal delay suggesting that growth hormone is more important than thyroid.
- Maxilla and mandible are affected → leading to malocclusion in pituitary dwarfs.

- Have a low caries rate due to longer period of maturation and delayed eruption. When over activity of pituitary occurs after puberty, growth of mandible occurs → projection of chin.
- Supraeruption to teeth → overgrowth of the alveolar process → increased size of the dental arch → tongue becomes enlarged → Pronathism.

INFLUENCE OF PARATHYROID HORMONE

Enamel formed after the removal of parathyroid gland shows opaque areas and some spots without the usual yellow pigment.

Enamel organ → disorganized and broken down into epithelial cysts → shortening of ameloblasts.

Immediate affects on the dentin → Marked caleiotraumatic line followed by a zone of hypomineralized dentin. Later effects → more variable.

- Fractures of the teeth at weak spots in the dentin → frequently found.

Effect of parathyroid disease when the teeth are mineralizing are an → exaggeration of incremental lines → minor alterations of fairly normal bands of dentin and bands containing interglobular spaces.

Following changes occur in tissues forming during the PTH deficiency.

- Defects in matrix secretion and mineralization of enamel and dentin
- Delay in eruption
- Osteoclasts are less numerous → molar eruption cannot occur without bone resorption
- Loss of lamina dura
- Radiographs show that bones are osteoporoti with no change in the density of teeth
- Can cause malocclusion due to drifting of teeth.

INFLUENCE OF SEX HORMONES ON GINGIVAL AND ORAL MUCOSA FEMALE SEX HORMONES AND GONADOTROPHIC HORMONES

- Female sex hormones influence the growth of the oral epithelium
- They also dilate the blood vessels in the underlining tissue and increase their permeability.

GINGIVAL CHANGES RELATED TO MENSTRUATION

- Slight tendency for gingivitis to increase at puberty.
- Hormones affect preexisting inflammation but do not initiate it.

During Menstruation

Rise in concentration of bacterial hyaluronidase due to increase in bacterial numbers following the shedding of more epithelial cells.

Pregnancy Gingivitis

Increased permeability of blood vessels produced by progesterone and stimulation or oral epithelium by oestrogen sensitivity of the gingival to irritants is increased.

SEX DIFFERENCES ON DENTAL CARIES

Girls are more susceptible to caries than boys because teeth erupt at an earlier age in girls.
Therefore, the teeth are exposed to oral fluids for a longer period of time.

EFFECT OF ADRENAL STEROIDS AND SEX HORMONES ON THE SUPPORTING STRUCTURE OF THE TEETH

Cortisone and ACTH → favor osteoporosis in bone by interfering with the synthesis of new protein required in bone remodeling and accelerating the breakdown of existing bone matrix.

Androgens and pestrogens → inhibit the growth of bone but increase the size of trabecular which fuse forming a more solid bone with a smaller narrow cavity.

Ganglion

A mass of nervous tissue composed principally of nerve cell bodies and lying outside the brain on spinal cord serving as a center of energy from which nerve impulses are transmitted.

Trigeminal Ganglion
(Gasserian Ganglion or Semilunar Ganglious)

- This is the sensory ganglion of the fifth cranial nerve.
- It is made up of pseudounipolar nerve cells with 'T'-shaped arrangement of their process.
- The ganglion is *crescentic or semilunar* in shape with its convexity directed anterolaterally. The three divisions of trigeminal. Nerve emerge from this convexity.
- Posterior concavity of the ganglion receives the sensory root of the nerve.
- It occupies a special space of dura mater called the *Trigeminal or Meckel s cave.*

Relation Medially

Internal carotid artery posterior part of cavernous sinus

Laterally

Middle meningeal artery.

Superiority

Parahippocampal guys.

Inferiorly

Motor root of trigeminal nerve, greater petrosol nerve, apex of petrous temporal bone, foramen laresum.

ASSOCIATED ROOTS AND BRANCHES

- Central processes of the ganglion cells → sensory root of Trigeminal nerve.
- Peripheral processes of the ganglion cells → form 3 divisions of trigeminal N namely ophthalmic, maxillary and mandibular.
- Small motor root join the mandibular N.

Blood Supply

- Internal carotid
- Middle meningeal and
- Accessory meningeal arteries
- Meningeal branch of the ascending pharyngeal artery.

PARASYMPATHETIC GANGLIA

Submandibular Ganglion

Situation

Submandibular ganglion lies superficial to hyoglossus. M in the submandibular region. Functionally connected to facial nerve. Topographically connected to lingual branch of mandibular nerve.

Roots

1. Sensory root from lingual nerve.
2. Sympathetic root → sympathetic plexus around the facial artery.
3. Secretomotor root → from superior salivatory nucleus through nerves intermedius via chorda tympani which is a branch of facial nerve.

Branch

1. Direct branches to submandibular salivary gland.
2. Postganglionic fibers reach the sublingual salivary gland through the lingual nerve.

Pterygopalatine Ganglion (Sphenopalative Ganglion)

It is the largest parasympathetic ganglion suspended by roots.

Sensory: It is by the auriculotemporal nerve.

Sympathetic root: Sympathetic plexus around the middle meningeal artery.

Secretomotor roots: Fibers of lesser petrosal nerve relay in otic ganglion. Postganglionic fibers reach the parotid gland through auriculotemporal nerve.

Major roots: Branch from nerve to medial pterygoid.

Branches

Postganglionic branches of the ganglion pass through auriculotemporal nerve to supply the parotid gland.

Motor Branches
- Tensor veli palatine
- Tensor tympani

CILIARY GANGLION

- Very small ganglion present in the orbit. Topographically related to nasociliary. N functionally related to oculomotor nerve.
- It has no secretomotor fibers.

Roots

- *Sensory root* → is from long ciliary nerve.
- *Sympathetic root* → by long ciliary nerve from plexus around ophthalmic artery.
- *Motor root* – from a branch to inferior oblique muscle.
- *Branches:* Ganglion gives 10-12 short ciliary nerves containing postganglionic fibers for supply of constrictor or splinter pupillae and cilians muscle.

- Maxillary nerve, functionally related to facial nerve → Ganglion of Hay fever.

Roots

- *Sensory:* It is from maxillary nerve.
- *Sympathetic:* It is from postganglionic plexus around the internal carotid artery.
- *Secretomotor root:* It is from greater petrosal nerve which arises from geniculate ganglion of facial nerve.

Branches

1. *For lacrimal gland:* Postganglionic fibers pass → zygomatic branch of maxillary nerve lacrimal nerve → lacrimal gland.
2. *Nasopalatine nerve:* Supplies secretomotor fibers to both nasal and palatal glands.
3. *Palatine branches:* 2-3 lesser palatine branches → mucous and glands of soft membrane.
4. *Nasal branches:* Mucous membrane and lateral wall of nasal cavity.
5. *Orbital branches:* Orbital periosteum.
6. *Pharyngeal branches:* Glands of pharynx.

Otic Ganglion

Situation

Lies deep to the trunk of mandibular N between nerve and tensor veli palatini. M in the infratemporal fossa.

Functionally related to glossopharyngeal N topographically related to mandibular N.

Geniculate Ganglion

1. It is located on the first bend of the facial N in relation to the medial wall of middle ear.
2. It is a sensory ganglion.
3. The taste fibers present in the nerve are peripheral processes of pseudounipolan neurons present in the geniculate ganglion.

CRANIAL NERVES (FIGS 16.1 TO 16.6)

There are 12 pairs of cranial nerves which supply the muscles of eyeball, face, palate, pharynx, larynx, tongue and two large muscles of neck. Besides these are afferent to special senses like smell, sight, hearing, taste and touch.

TRIGEMINAL NERVE

It is the largest cranial nerve. The trigeminal is the 5th cranial nerve and it has three branches of which two are sensory and the 3rd is mixed.
1. Ophthalmic
2. Maxillary   Sensory
3. Mandibular – mixed

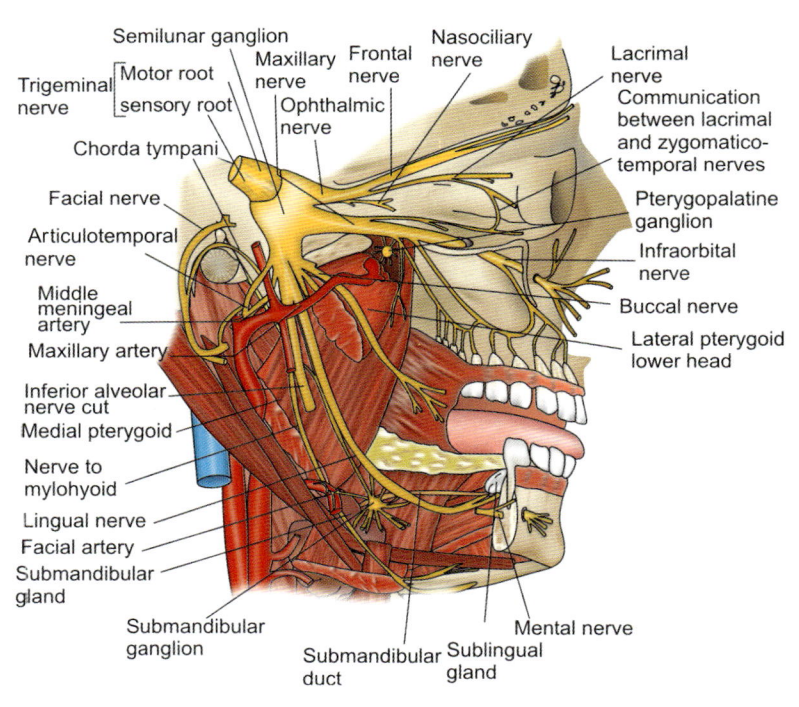

Fig. 16.1: Trigeminal nerve

Effects of Hormones on the Oral Structures

Table 16.1

Cranial nerve	Sensory (S) Motor (M) Mixed	Nuclei	Location	Function of the nerve component	Exit site
Olfactory (I)	Sensory			Sense of smell	Cribriform plate
Optic (II)	Sensory			Sight	Optic foramen
Occulumotor (III)	Motor	Oculomotor	Midbrain, level of superior colliculus	Movements of eyeball, contraction of pupil, accommodation proprioceptive	Superior orbital fissure
Trochlear (IV)	Motor	Abducent nucleus	Lower pens	Lateral movement of eyeball (proprioceptive)	Superior orbital fissure
Vestibulo cohlear (VII)	Sensory				
Cochlear		Two cochlear nuclei dorsal and ventral	Junction of medulla and pens	Hearing equilibrium of head	Internal acoustic (auditory) meatus
Vestibular		Four vestibular nuclei superior, spinal, medial and lateral			

Contd[a]

Contd[a]

Cranial nerve	Sensory (S) Motor (M) Mixed	Nuclei	Location	Function of the nerve component	Exit site
Vagus (X) and Cranial part of XI N	Mixed (sensory and motor)	Nucleus ambiguous dorsal nucleus of Vagus nucleus of tractus solitatius	Medulla	Movement of palate, pharynx and larynx motor and secretomotor to bronchial tree and gut, inhibitory to heart. Sensations from viscera taste from post most tongue and epidlothis. Sensations from the skin of external ear go to the spinal nucleus of V nerve	Jugular foramen
Spinal Accessory (II)	Motor	Spinal nucleus of accessory nerve	Spinal wrd, C1-5	Sternocleidomastoid and Trapesius	Jugular foramen

OPHTHALMIC NERVE

This is the first branch of Trigeminal N. From the convexity of the trigeminal ganglion, it runs in the lateral wall of cavernous sinus below the broacher and above the maxillary division.

At the anterior end of the sinus, it divides into 3 branches.
- Nasociliary
- Frontal
- Lacrimal

I. OPHTHALMIC NERVE

Sensory

Nasociliary

Course and relative: It enters the orbit by passing through the superior orbital fissure within tendinous arch and between the two division of oculomotor.

In the orbit: Along with ophthalmic A it crosses the medial wall of orbit above the optic N and below the superior Rectus M. Its terminal part continues as anterior ethmoid nerve.

BRANCHES AND DISTRIBUTION

1. Sensory branches → skin of nose mucous membrane of nose in its roof.
2. Long ciliary nerve (2 to 3) → convey postganglionic sympathetic fibers to dialator pupillae. Sensory to Iris cornea, ciliary body.
3. Infratrochlear nerve → sensory to skin of cyclids, nasal skin above angle of eye.
4. Posterior ethmoidal nerve → supplies ethmoidal and sphenoidal sinuses.
5. Branch to ciliary ganglion.
6. Anterior ethmoidal
    - Internal nasal
    - External nasal

7. *Frontal:* Supraorbital (to prehead, scalp as far as vertex upper cyclid, frontal sinus).

   Supratrochlear (to skin of medial part of forehead and medial part of upper eyelid).

   Lacrimal: (To lacinal gland, skin of lateral part of upper eyelid, conjunctiva).

MAXILLARY NERVE

This is 2nd branch of trigeminal nerve. It is entirely sensory and arises from the convexity of trigeminal ganglion.

COURSE

- The nerve runs forwards in the lower angle of the lateral wall of cavernous sinus.
- It leaves the cranial cavity through foramen rotundum.
- After traversing pterygopalatine fossa, it enters the orbit through the inferior orbital fissure.
- In the orbit, it runs as **infraorbital nerve** in infraorbital groove and **infraorbital canal**.
- It emerges on the face through infraorbital foramen.

RELATIONS

a. *In the cranial cavity:* It lies in the lower angle of the lateral wall of cavernous sinus. Above it is ophthalmic nerve Lateral—Temporal lobe, Medial to it—Internal carotid A and abducent N.

b. *In the pterygopalatine fossa:* It lies close to the terminal part of the maxillary artery.

BRANCHES

a. *Intracranial:* Meningeal to dura of middle cranial fossa.
b. In the pterygopalatine fossa divides
   - Zygomaticotemporal (skin of anterior temporal communicating branch to region) lacrimal nerve
   - Zygomalicofacial (skin over zygomatic bone).

Effects of Hormones on the Oral Structures 165

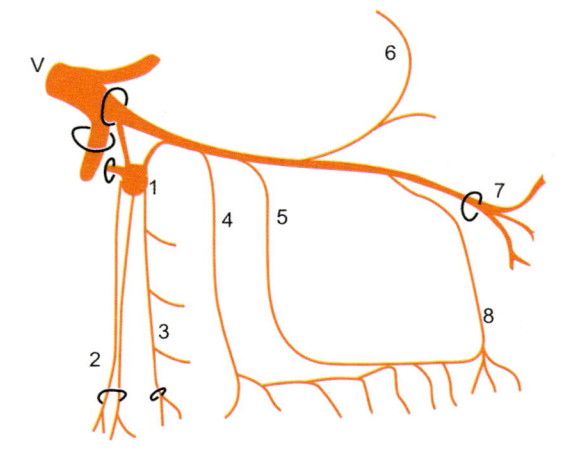

1. Pterygopalatine ganglion
2. Lesser palatine nerves
3. Greater palatine nerve
4. Posterior superior alveolar nerve
5. Middle superior alveolar nerve
6. Zygomaticotemporal branch of zygomatic nerve
7. Infraorbital nerve
8. Anterior superior alveolar nerve

Fig. 16.2: Maxillary nerve

c. *Ganglion branches:* There are two from which pterygopalatine ganglion is suspended. The sensory branches pass through the ganglion without relay to supply nasal cavity. The branches of the ganglion are actually branches of maxillary nerve. They are:
  i. *Orbital branches*
   – Supply periosteum of orbit and orbitalis muscle.
  ii. *Palatine branches*
   – Greater palatine nerve—supplies hard palate and lateral wall of the nose.

- Lesser (or) middle and posterior palatine supply the soft palate and tonsil.
  iii. *Nasal branches*
    - Lateral posterior superior nasal (6 in No.) – Post parts of superior and middle contralateral.
    - Medical posterior superior nasal nerves – Posterior part of roof of nose and nasal septum. Largest of these nerves – Nasopalatine nerve which descends upto anterior Part of hard palate through the incisive foramen.
  iv. Pharyngeal branch – supplier part of thenasopharynx behind the auditory tube.
  v. Lacrimal branch – supply lacrimal gland.
  vi. Posterior superior alveolar branch – (gingival cheek and molar teeth, maxillary sinus).

Infraorbital Nerve

- *Middle superior alveolar* – maxillary sinus supplier, upper premolar teeth.
- *Anterior superior alveolar* – upper incisor canine teeth, maxillary sinus anterior inferior part of nasal cavity.
- *Terminal branch* – Palpebral, Nasal, Labial.

MANDIBULAR NERVE

Third and posttraumatic branch of trigeminal nerve.

Origin

From the convex border of trigeminal ganglion in the middle cranial fossa. It is a mixed nerve.

Course

The nerve passes through formen Ovale and enters infratemporal fossa. Here it divides into an anterior and posterior division.

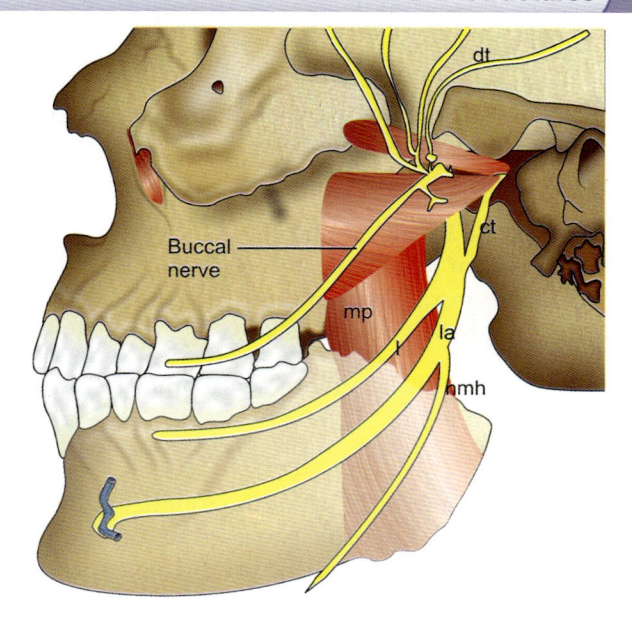

Fig. 16.3: Mandibular nerve

Relations

1. In the foramen ovale. Nerve lies along with:
    i. Accessory meningeal artery
    ii. *Emissary vein* – which connects pterygoid plexus to cavernous sinus.
2. In the infratemporal fossa. The nerve is related to:
    i. *Medially* – otic ganglion, tensor palate M.
    ii. *Laterally* – Lateral Pterygoid M.
    iii. *Posterior* – Middle meningeal A.

Branches

- From main trunk.
- Meningeal branch to dura in middle cranial fossa.
- Nerve to medial pterygoid also supplies tensor tympani and T. palatil.
    - Nerve to lateral pterygoid.
    - Anterior and posterior deep temporal nerves to temporalis nerve.

Anterior Division
- Nerve to masseter.
- *Buccal nerve* – supplier skin over buccinator and the mucous membrane on its inner surface.

Posterior Division
- It passes medial to lateral pterygoid.
- Auriculo (skin of tragiono).
- Superficial temporal (skin of temple).

Auriculotemporal
- Secretomotor to parotid gland (secretomotor and sensory).
- Articular to TM joint.

Lingual
- Sensory to the anterior 2/3rd of the tongue and to the floor of mouth. Fibers of chorda tympani secretomotor to the submandibular and sublingual salivary glands and gustatory to ant. 2/3rds of the tongue, are also distributed through lingual nerve.
- Larger terminal branch of the post in of mandibular nerve.
- *Mylohyoid branch* – supplies mylohyoid M and ant. Belly of diagnostic.

Inferior Alveolar Nerve
- While running in mandibular canal, gives branches that supply teeth and gums.
- Incisive branch.
- Mental nerve.

Mental N
Emerges at the mental foramen and supplies skin of chin and the skin and mucous membrane of the lower lip.

Incisive Branch
Supplies the labial aspect of gums of canine and incisor teeth.

FACIAL NERVE (VII N)
Facial nerve is a mixed nerve whose functional components and connected nuclei are listed below.

Effects of Hormones on the Oral Structures

It supplies all the muscles of facial expression developed from 2nd pharyngeal/branchial arch. Its various nuclear components are:

	Special visceral efferent	General visceral efferent	Special visceral afferent	General somatic afferent
Supplies	Muscles of facial expression	Lacrimal, nasal, palatal, pharyngeal glands through greater petrosal nerve submandibular and sublingual salivary gland through chorda tympani nerve	Raisins taste fibers from anterior 2/3rds of tongue except circum vallate papillae and general visceral afferent from various glands	Priopriceptive fibers from muscles of facial expression
Nucleus	Is at lower pons	Are lacrimatory and superior salivatory	Tractus solitarius	Spinal nucleus of VCN

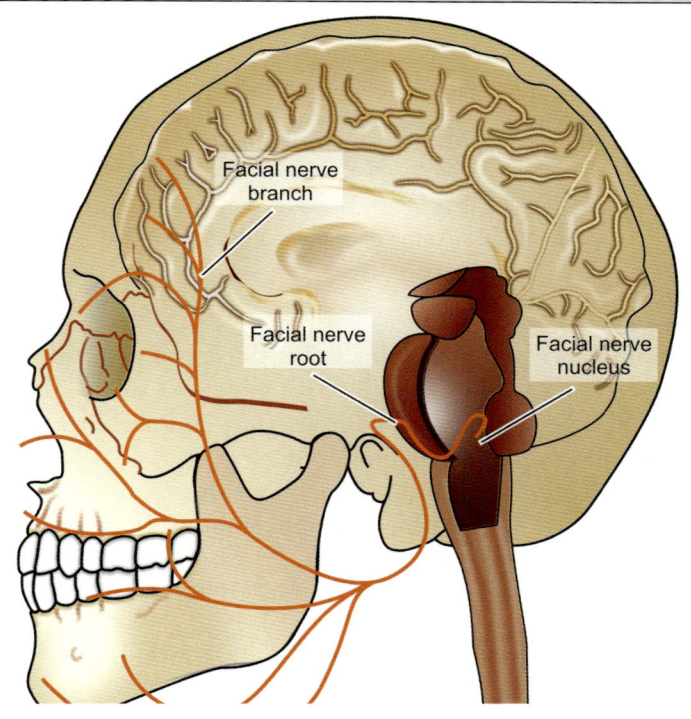

Fig. 16.4A: Facial nerve

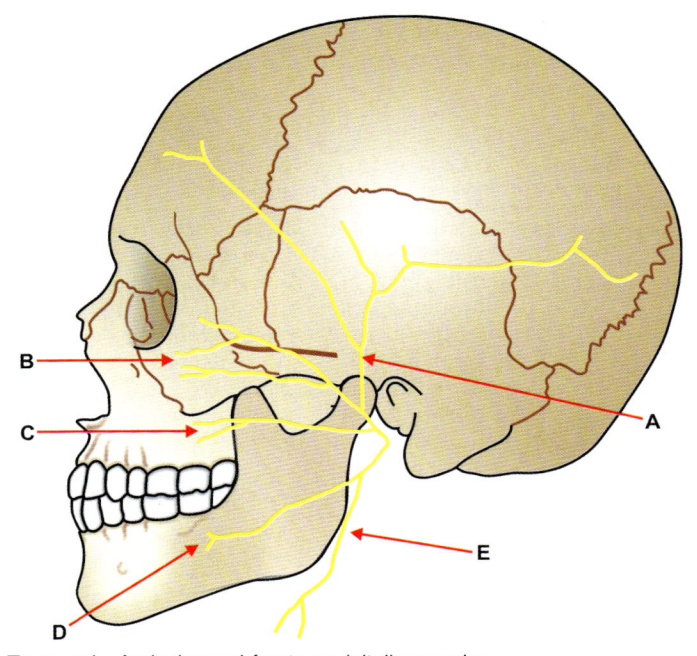

170 Oral Physiology

A. Temporal—Auricular and fronto-occipitalis muscles
B. Zygomatic—Muscles of the zygomatic arch and orbit
C. Buccal—Muscles in the cheek and above the mouth
D. Mandibular—Muscle in the region of the mandible
E. Cervical—Platysma muscle

Fig. 16.4B: Terminal branches of facial nerve

COURSE

The main nerve emerges at the lower border of pons above the olive.
- The nerves intermedius composed of 2nd and 3rd nuclear components join the main nerve.
- These two enter internal acoustic meatus.
- They run laterally in the petrous temporal bone where the two fuse to form a single trunk.
- It forms a bend, which is enlarged to form geniculate ganglion.
- It runs posteriorly in the medial wall of middle ear.

Effects of Hormones on the Oral Structures — 171

- Finally it curves downwards traversing the facial canal.
- Lastly, the nerve exists through the cranial cavity by passing through the stylomastoid foramen as purely motor nerve.

INTRACRANIAL BRANCHES

1. *Through geniculate ganglion:* Greater petrusol nerve (from nerves intermedius) joins with deep petrosal (sympathetic fibers) to form nerve of pterygoid canal.
2. *N to the stapedius as it traverse facial canal:* Supplies stapedius M.
3. *Chorda tympani N:* Secretomotor fibers to submandibular and sublingual salivary gland. Taste fibers to ant. 2/3rd of tongue.

EXTRACRANIAL COURSE

All the exit of stylomastoid foramen.
1. *Posterior auricular brand:* Supplies auriculasis posterior, occipitalis, intrinsic muscles on the back of the auricle.
2. *Stylohyoid branch:* Supplies stylohyoid M.
3. *Digastric branch:* Supplies digastric M.

In the Parotid Gland

- *Temporal branches:* Supply frontalis part of ouipitofrontalis M.
- *Zygomatic branches:* Orbicularis oculi.
- *Buccal branches:* Bufeinator, muscles of nose and upper lip.
- *Marginal mandibular:* Lower lip and chin.
- *Cervical branch:* Platysna.

GLOSSOPHARYNGEAL NERVE

It is the ninth cranial nerve. It is a mixed nerve nuclear columns/ functional components:

Oral Physiology

	Special visceral efferent	General visceral efferent	General visceral afferent and special visceral afferent	General somatic afferent
Supplies	One muscle stylopharyngeus	Parotid salivary gland after relay in otic ganglion	General sensation from post 1/3rd of tongue, tonsil, pharynx, carotid body, carotid sinus. Taste-post 1/3rd of tongue and vallate papillae	Prioprioceptive impulses from (pharyngeal M)
Nucleus	Nucleus	Inferior salivatory nucle	Nucleus of Tracitus solitarius	Nucleus of spinal tract of Trigeminal N

INTRACRANIAL COURSE

- Fibers of nerve arise from respective nuclear columns at the level of Medulla oblongata.
- It passes between olive and inferior cebellar peduncle.
- It is attached at the base of brain in the posteriolateral sulius between olive and inferior cerebellar peduncle by 3-4 rootlets.
- The rootlets join to form the nerve which enters the middle part of the jugular foramen in a separate sheath of dura mater.

Effects of Hormones on the Oral Structures 173

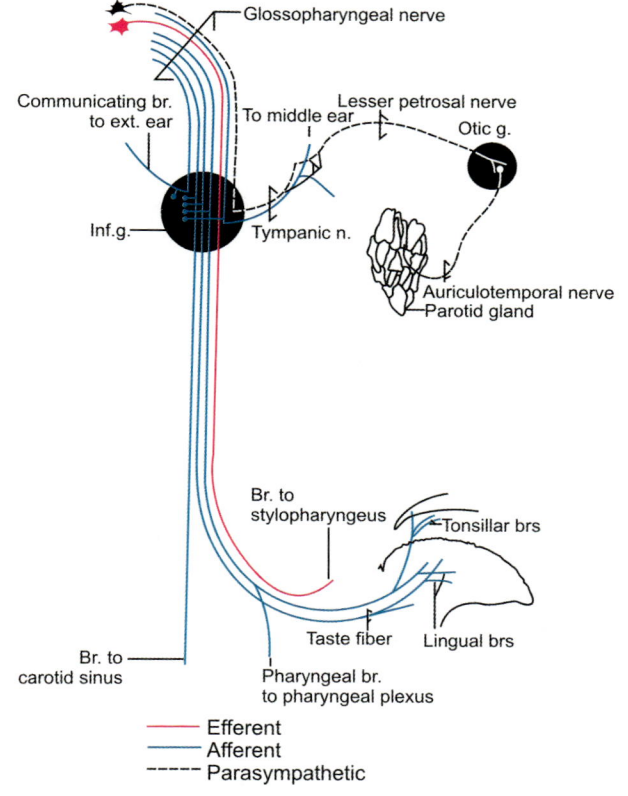

Fig. 16.5: Glossopharyngeal nerve

EXTRACRANIAL COURSE

- Superior ganglion is small and is a detached part of the inferior ganglion.
- The inferior ganglion is larger and its central processes carry the sensory fibers to the nerve (general and special sensation).
- It curves medially across the stylopharyngeus M and supplies it.
- It enters the pharynx through the interval between superior and middle constrictor muscles and ends by dividing into its terminal branches.

BRANCHES

1. Motor to stylopharyngeus M.
2. *Tympanic branch:* Contributes to tympanic plexus from where branches are given to
   a. Pharyngotympanic tube
   b. Middle ear
   c. Lesser petrosal N.
3. *Carotid branch:* This descends on the internal carotid A to supply carotid body and the carotid sinus.
4. *Pharyngeal branch:* Joins with pharyngeal branch of Vagus and superior cervical ganglion to form the pharyngeal plexus.
5. *Tonsillar branches:* Supply tonsil and Oropharynx
6. *Lingual branches:* Conveys taste and ordinary sensation from posterior 1/3 of tongue.

BRANCHES OF COMMUNICATION

1. Communicating branches are with vagus and superior cervical sympathetic ganglion.

HYPOGLOSSAL NERVE

The hypoglossal N is the twelfth cranial nerve. It is motor in function (Somatic efferent) and supplies all the muscles of the tongue except palatoglossus.

ORIGIN

- Its nucleus is situated in the medulla in the floor of IV ventricle deep to hypoglossal triangle.

COURSE OF THE NERVE

- The rootlets are attached in the groove between the pyramid and olive.

Effects of Hormones on the Oral Structures 175

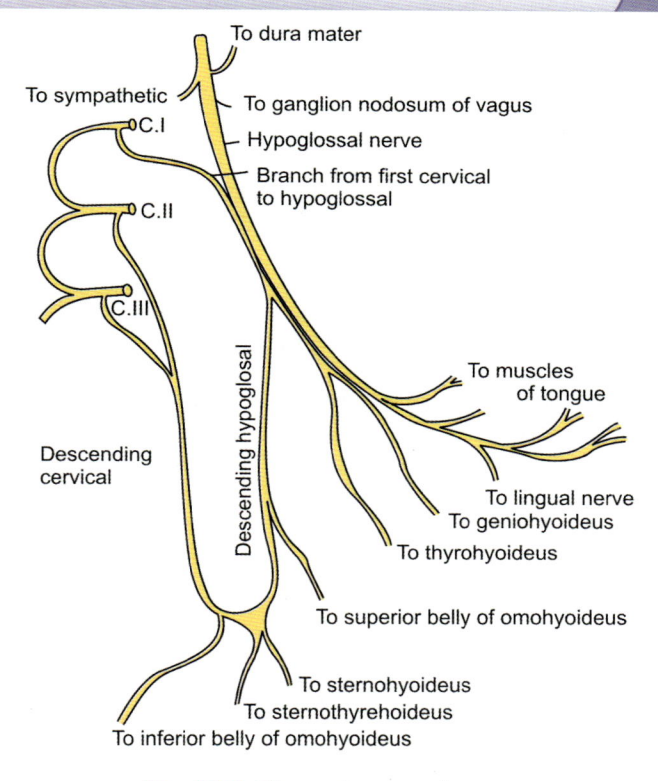

Fig. 16.6: Glossopharyngeal nerve

- The rootlets join the form two bundles which pierce the dura mater separately near the anterior condylav canal or hypoglossal canal.
- It enters the neck through anterior condylar canal and decends between internal jugular V and internal carolett.
- It curves around the vagus N.
- It makes a wide curve crossing the internal carolid external carotid and loop of lingual A.
- It passes above the hyoid bone in the submandibular region, superficial to hyoglossus where it ends by dividing into its muscular branches.

BRANCHES

Of communication with Vagus, ventral ramus of I carnival N, lingual N and superior cervical ganglion of sympathetic chain of distribution.

Extrinsic muscles of tongue	Intrinsic muscles of tongue
Styloglossus	Superior longitudinal
Genioglossus	Inferior longitudinal
Hyoglossus	Transverse muscle
	Vertical muscle

Carries fibers of ventral ramus of I cervical which gets distributed as—Meningeal branch, Superior limb of ansa cervicalis, Branch to thyrohyoid and geniohyoid muscles.

Role of Calcium

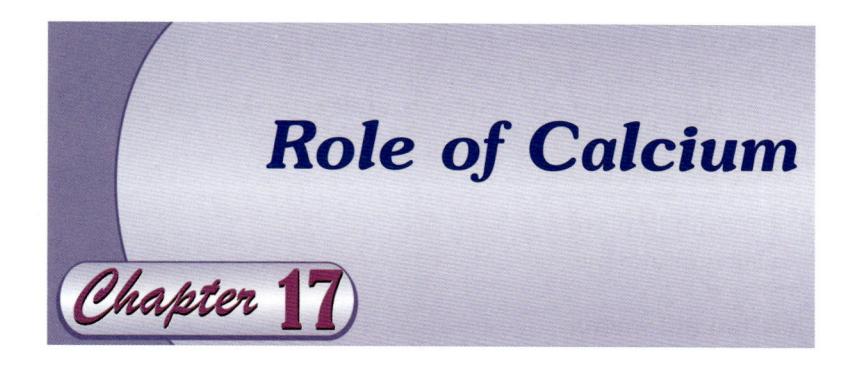

Chapter 17

INTRODUCTION

Calcium is an important, inorganic ion for many physiological functions. Calcium is very essential for many activities in the body such as:
1. Neuronal activity
2. Skeletal muscle activity
3. Cardiac activity
4. Smooth muscle activity
5. Secretory activity of the glands
6. Coagulation of blood

In the bones and teeth, 90% of the body calcium is present and test is present in the plasma.

SOURCE

 i. Milk
 ii. Dairy products like cheese and butter
 iii. Egg
 iv. Meat
 v. Fish
 vi. Wheat

NORMAL VALUE

- In a normal young healthy adult, there is about 1100 g of calcium in the body.

- It forms about 1.5% of total body weight.
- Normal blood calcium is 9.4 mg% range ⇒ (9-11 mg%).
- The requirement of calcium in adult is 0.7-1.00 gm per day.

TYPES OF CALCIUM

a. Calcium in plasma
b. Calcium in bone

Calcium in Plasma

- Normal level is 9-11 mg% (5 mg/lit or 2.5 mml/lit)
- It exists in 3 forms
  − Ionized (40%)
  − Bound (40-50%)
  − Complex (10%)
- The ionized calcium is the one which gives the physiological effects. The bound form of calcium is attached to the plasma protein, albumin and globulin, while the complex form is the result of calcium combining with the anions like phosphates, sulphates and oxalates.

ABSORPTION OF CALCIUM

- About 1000 mg of calcium is taken in diet daily and out of it 300 mg is absorbed in the upper part of the small incentive.
- Both passive and active transport are involved in this process.
- The active transport is facilitated by 1,25-dihydroxy cholecalciferol, which is a meta belief of Vit 'D' produced in the kidneys.
- Calcium absorption is inhibited by phosphates, oxalates and alkalis as they form invaluable calcium salts in the intestine.
- Calcium is also secreted in the digestive juices (125 mg/day). Daily Ca^{++} absorption in the body will be 175 mg.

Role of Calcium 179

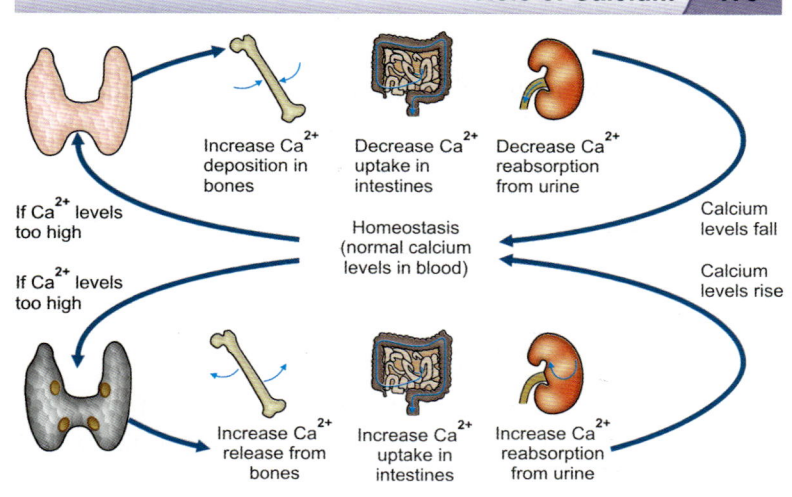

Fig. 17.1: Calcium regulation

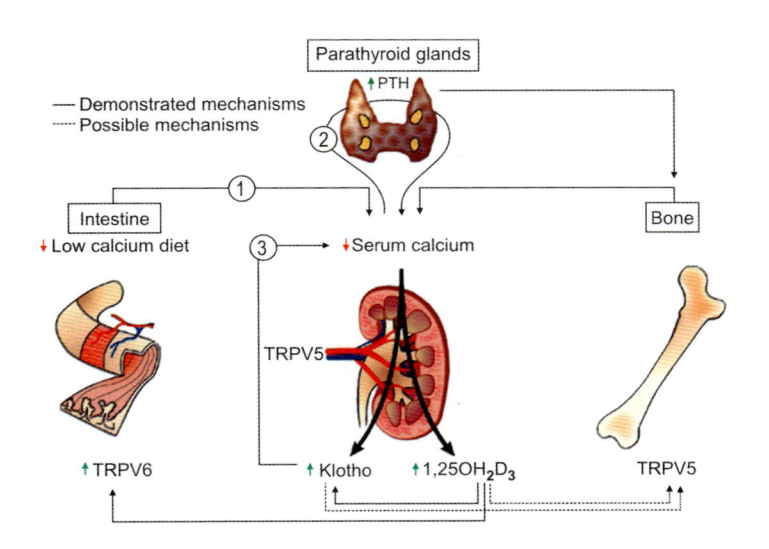

If Ca²⁺ levels too high → Increase Ca²⁺ deposition in bones → Decrease Ca²⁺ uptake in intestines → Decrease Ca²⁺ reabsorption from urine → Calcium levels fall → Homeostasis (normal calcium levels in blood)

If Ca²⁺ levels too high → Increase Ca²⁺ release from bones → Increase Ca²⁺ uptake in intestines → Increase Ca²⁺ reabsorption from urine → Calcium levels rise → Homeostasis (normal calcium levels in blood)

Fig. 17.2: Calcium regulation

— Demonstrated mechanisms
----- Possible mechanisms

Parathyroid glands ↑PTH

Intestine — ↓Low calcium diet — ↑TRPV6

↓Serum calcium

TRPV5

↑Klotho   ↑1,25OH$_2$D$_3$

Bone — TRPV5

Calcium in Bone

- As mentioned earlier, the plasma calcium level ranges from 9-11 mg%. About 50% of this is deposited and resorbed from the bone.
- The calcium in bones is present as inorganic salts of hydroxyapatites. It is essential that adequate quantities of matrix and salts of hydroxyapatites are present to ensure normal bone structure.

CALCIUM EXCRETION

- Most of the calcium, which is filtered in the kidneys is reabsorbed in the proximal tubules, thick ascending limb of the loop of Henle and distal renal tubules.
- In the distal tubule, the absorption of calcium is regulated by the parathyroid hormone.
- The amount of calcium excreted in the crine is equal to the net amount of calcium absorbed from the gut.
- The unabsorbed calcium in the intestines together with the calcium secreted by the digestive juices is excreted in the faces.

CALCIUM REGULATION

- Three hormones play an important role in calcium metabolism.
- They are parathyroid hormone, calcitonin and 1,25-dihydroxy cholecalciferol.
- Metabolism is also affected by certain other hormones like growth hormone, cortisol, estrogen and growth factors.

FUNCTIONS

- Formation and growth of bones and teeth
- Blood coagulation
- For the action of intracellular enzymes
- Transmission of nerve impulse
- Neurotransmitter release

Role of Calcium 181

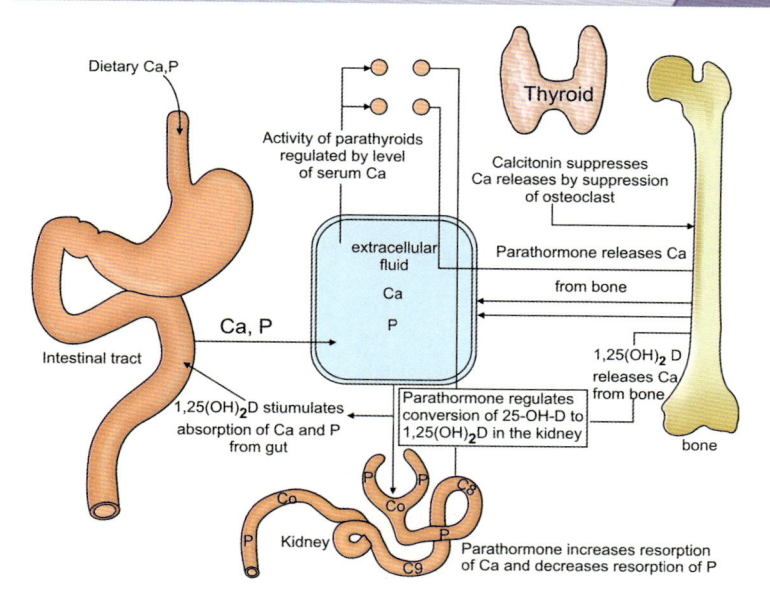

Fig. 17.3: Calcium regulation

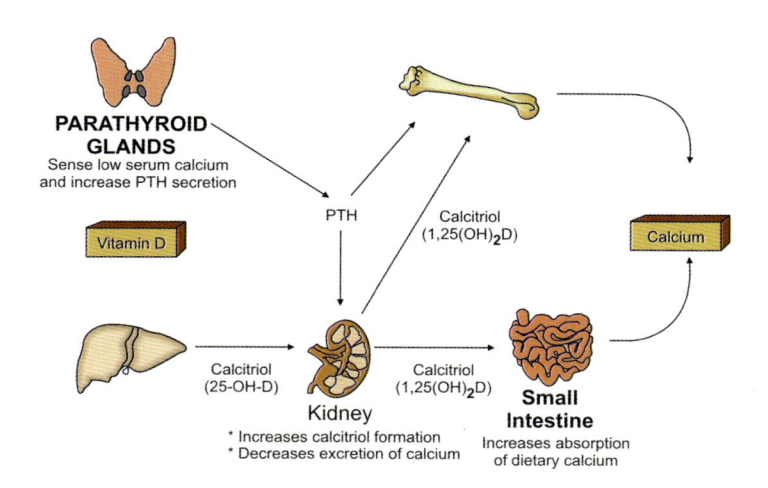

Fig. 17.4: Calcium regulation

- Excitation—contraction coupling in muscle
- Contraction of muscles
- Secretion of hormones
- Act as second messenger for hormone action.

Section 3

Dental Anatomy

Introduction of Dentition

Chapter 18

INTRODUCTION

Teeth form the most important component of the oral cavity.

In non-mammalian vertebrates the teeth are constantly replaced throughout life, a condition called polyphyodonty. But most mammalians has two sets of erupting phase called diphyodonty. Usually these two sets of erupting phase to be known as primary or deciduous which are replaced later by permanent dentition.

A tooth in man consists of three hard tissues, the enamel, dentin and cementum, surrounding a soft tissue—the pulp. The part covered by enamel is known as crown and the part covered by cementum is root. The line of junction of the crown and the root is known as cemento-enamel junction or cervical line.

On the basis of fovin and function, the human teeth may be divided into three classes in case of primary dentition (incisor, canine and molar) and four classes in case of permanent dentition, i.e. (incisor, canine, premolars and molars).

The dentition can be divided into three period of stage.
1. Primary dentition – lasting from 6 months to 6 years
2. Mixed dentition – 6 years to 13 years
3. Permanent dentition – lasting from 13 years onwards.

There are 20 deciduous teeth and 32 permanent teeth to be noted.

Dental Anatomy

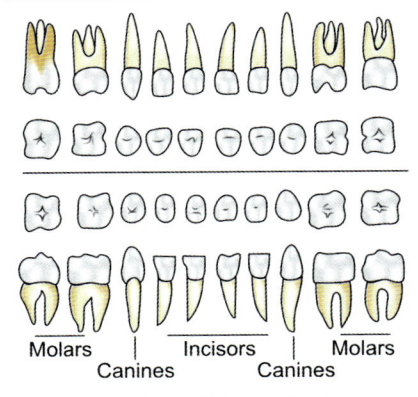

Fig. 18.1: Primary teeth

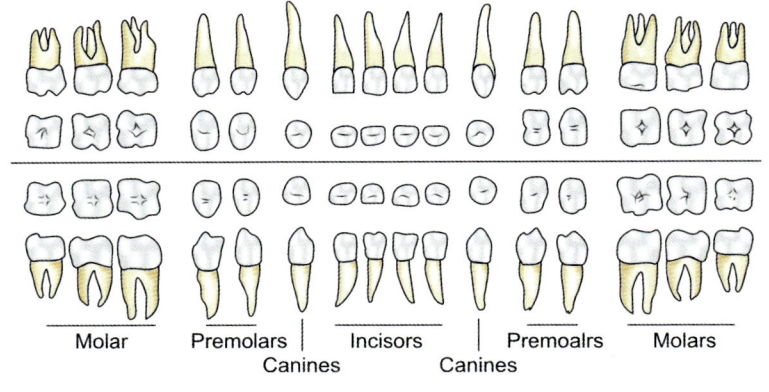

Fig. 18.2: Primary teeth

The teeth are arranged in two dental arches—1. Maxillary or upper arch, 2. Mandibular or lower arch. They are further classified into four quadrants where each quadrant will have 5 deciduous and 8 permanent tooth of either right or left quadrant.

FUNCTIONS OF TEETH

1. Helps in mastication
2. Aids in articulation and speech
3. Gives shape and beauty to the face

Introduction of Dentition

4. Like in animals, it may be used for self protection and attack. The human detail formula is as follows:
   Deciduous – DI 2/2   DC 1/1   DM 2/2
   Permanent – I 2/2   C 1/1   P 2/2   M 3/3

TOOTH SURFACES

The central incisors, lateral incisors, canines are collectively called as Anterior teeth.

The premolars and molar teeth are collectively known as posterior teeth.

The surfaces are as follows:
1. Labial surface   – It is the surface facing the lips.
2. Buccal surface   – It is the surface of teeth facing the cheeks.
3. Facial surface   – Buccal and labial surfaces are collectively known as facial surface.
4. Lingual surface – Surface of tooth present towards tongue.
5. Proximal surface – Surface of tooth with the adjacent teeth in the same dental arch. It has again two surfaces mesial and distal.
6. Occlusal surface – Surface that contacts opposing teeth is called occlusal surface.
7. Incisal surface – It is the cutting edge of anterior teeth, analogus to the occlusal surface of the posterior teeth.

LANDMARKS

Cusp – It is a prominent elevation on the occlusal surface of a posterior tooth.

Cingulum – It is a bulbous convexity formed in the cervical third of the lingual surface of the anterior teeth.

Tubercle – It is a small elevation that may be found on same portion of the crown. They are usually formed by addition of enamel.

188 Dental Anatomy

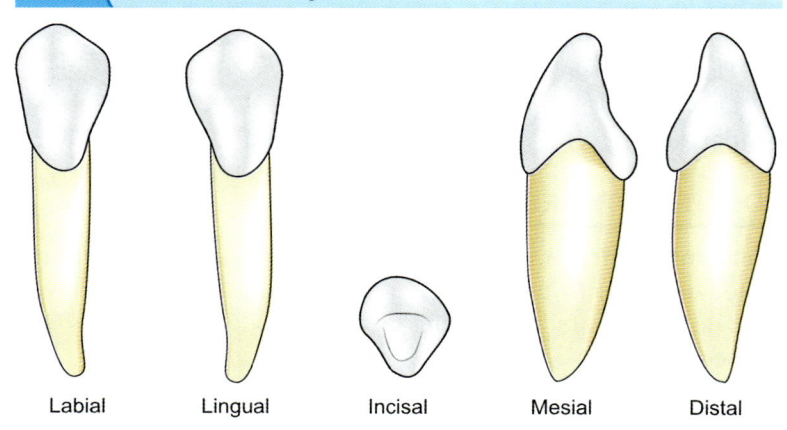

Fig. 18.3: Mandibular right permanent canine

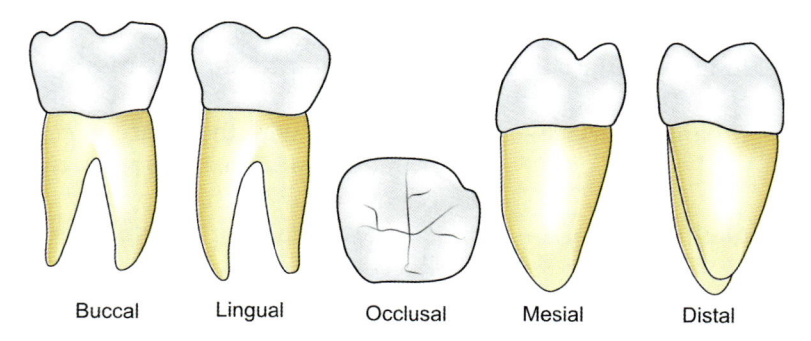

Labial Lingual Incisal Mesial Distal

Fig. 18.4: Mandibular right first permanent molar

Buccal Lingual Occlusal Mesial Distal

Ridge — It is a linear elevation on the surface of the tooth.

Marginal ridge — It is a linear elevation found at the mesial and distal edge of occlusal surface of posterior teeth. In case of incisors and canines, the marginal ridges form on the mesial, and distal ridges form on the mesial and distal margins of the lingual surface.

Introduction of Dentition 189

Fissure	– It is a long cleft between cusps or ridges.
Fossa	– It is a rounded depression on the surface of the tooth.
Triangular Fossa	– They are depressions formed mesial and distal to the marginal ridges on the occlusal surface of posterior teeth.
Sulcus	– It is a long depression on the surface of a tooth between ridges or cusps.
Developmental groove	– It is a groove or line formed between the primary parts of the crown or root. Buccal and lingual grooves are developmental grooves formed on the buccal and lingual surfaces of posterior teeth.
Pits	– They are minute depressions located at the junction of grooves or at their termination.
Lobe	– It is one of the primary sections of formation in the development of crown. The cusps of posterior teeth and mamelons of anterior teeth represents the lobe.
Cervical margin	– It is the junction of the anatomica crown and the anatomical root.
Oblique ridge	– It crosses obliquely the occlusal surface of maxillary molars. It is favored by the union of the triangular ridge of the distobuccal cusps and the distal ridge of the mesiolingual cusp.
Triangular ridge	– Descending cuspal tips of molars and premolars towards the central part of the occlusal surface.
Transverse ridge	– A transverse ridge is the union of two triangular ridges crossing transversely the surface of a posterior tooth.

LINE ANGLES AND POINT ANGLES

Line angles and point angles are used in order to aid in description of a tooth.

Line Angle

It is a union of two surfaces.

Line Angles for Anterior Teeth

There are 6 line angles therefore:
1. Mesiolabial
2. Distolabial
3. Mesiolingual
4. Distolingual
5. Labioincisal
6. Linguoincisal

Line Angles for Posterior Teeth

There are 8 line angles for the posterior tooth, they are:
1. Mesiobuccal
2. Distobuccal
3. Mesiolingual
4. Distolingual
5. Mesio-occlusal
6. Disto-occlusal
7. Bucco-occlusal
8. Linguo-occlusal

Point Angles

They are formed by union of 3 surfaces.

Point Angles for Anterior Teeth

There are 4 point angles for anterior teeth they are:
1. Mesiolabio incisal
2. Distolabio incisal
3. Mesiolingual incisal
4. Distolingual incisal

Introduction of Dentition

Point Angles for Posterior Teeth

There are 4 point angles for posterior teeth, they are:
1. Mesiobucco occlusal
2. Distobucco occlusal
3. Mesiolinguo occlusal
4. Distolinguo occlusal

TOOTH NUMBERING SYSTEMS

In order to help in identification of teeth, a system of tooth designation or tooth numbering is essential. The followings are some commonly used systems.

FDI Systems

A two digit nomenclature system was proposed by the Federation Dentaire Internationale in 1971. It is been adopted by WHO and International Association for Dental Research.

Each tooth is given two digits. The first digit indicates the quadrant while the second digit indicates the tooth in the quadrant. This system can be used for both permanent and deciduous teeth. Since this system is very easy to access in computers it is been widely used in all over the world.

For Permanent Dentition

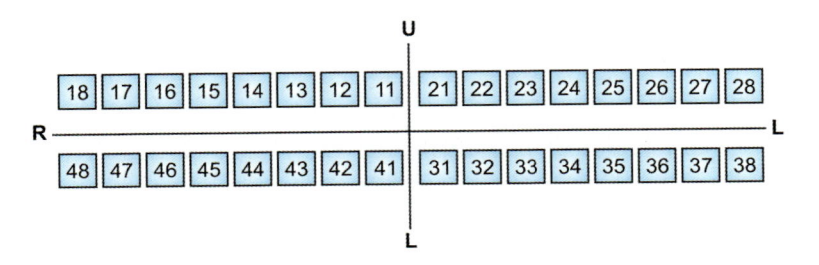

```
                            U
   18 17 16 15 14 13 12 11 | 21 22 23 24 25 26 27 28
R ─────────────────────────┼───────────────────────── L
   48 47 46 45 44 43 42 41 | 31 32 33 34 35 36 37 38
                            L
```

Fig. 18.5

192 Dental Anatomy

For Deciduous Dentition

```
              U
 55 54 53 52 51 | 61 62 63 64 65
R ─────────────────────────────── L
 85 84 83 82 81 | 71 72 73 74 75
              L
```

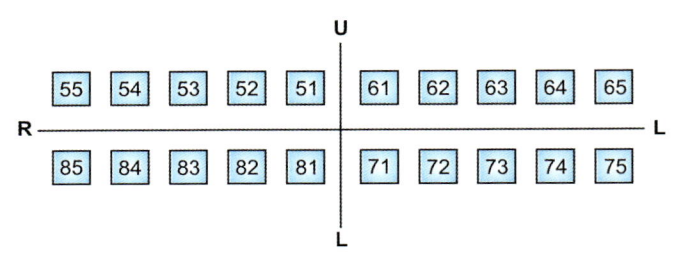

Fig. 18.6

Universal System

The American Dental Association put forward this tooth notation system.

For Permanent Dentition

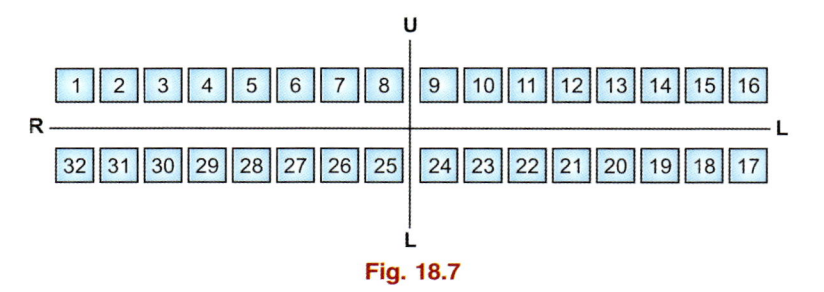

```
                    U
 1  2  3  4  5  6  7  8 | 9  10 11 12 13 14 15 16
R ──────────────────────────────────────────────── L
 32 31 30 29 28 27 26 25| 24 23 22 21 20 19 18 17
                    L
```

Fig. 18.7

For Deciduous Dentition

```
              U
 A  B  C  D  E | F  G  H  I  J
R ─────────────────────────────── L
 T  S  R  Q  P | O  N  M  L  K
              L
```

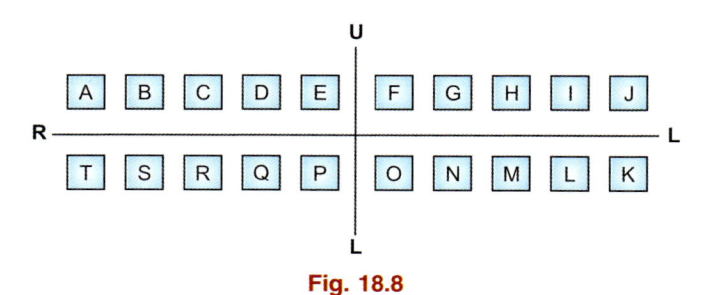

Fig. 18.8

Zsigmondy/Palmar Notation

This is a grid system of tooth designation described in 1861.

For Permanent Dentition

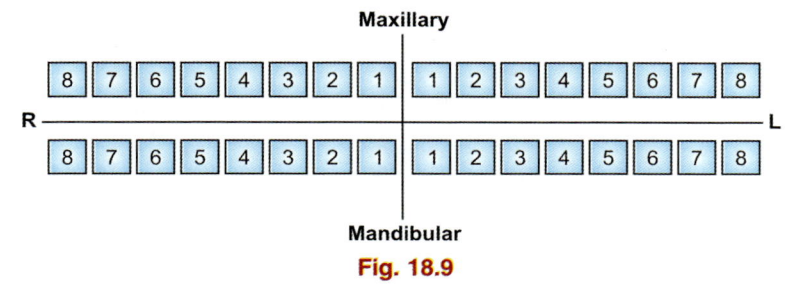

Maxillary

R | 8 | 7 | 6 | 5 | 4 | 3 | 2 | 1 | 1 | 2 | 3 | 4 | 5 | 6 | 7 | 8 | L

| 8 | 7 | 6 | 5 | 4 | 3 | 2 | 1 | 1 | 2 | 3 | 4 | 5 | 6 | 7 | 8 |

Mandibular

Fig. 18.9

For Deciduous Dentition

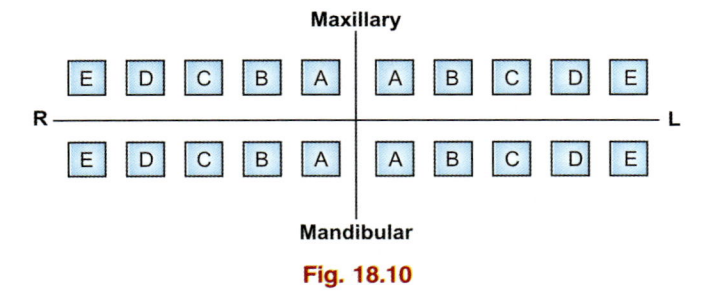

Maxillary

R | E | D | C | B | A | A | B | C | D | E | L

| E | D | C | B | A | A | B | C | D | E |

Mandibular

Fig. 18.10

TOOTH MORPHOLOGY OF PRIMARY DENTITION AND DIFFERENCE BETWEEN PRIMARY AND SECONDARY DENTITION

THE PRIMARY DENTITION

Introduction

The primary teeth are also called "milk", "temporary" and "baby" teeth. The primary teeth are later replaced by the permanent teeth. The primary teeth are twenty in number, five in each of the quadrants.

Dental Anatomy

Table 18.1: Chronology of the human primary dentition

Tooth	Hard tissue	Amount of enamel formed at birth	Enamel completed	Eruption	Root completed
Primary dentition					
Maxillary					
Central incisor	4 mon. in utero	Five sixths	1½ mon.	7½ mon.	1½ years
Lateral incisor	4½ mon. in utero	Two thirds	2½ mon.	9 mon.	2 years
Cuspid	5 mon. in utero	One third	9 mon.	18 mon.	3¼ years
First molar	5 mon. in utero	Cusps united	6 mon.	14 mon.	2½ years
Second molar	6 mon. in utero	Cusp tips still isolated	11 mon.	24 mon.	3 years
Mandibular					
Central incisor	4½ mon. in utero	Three fifths	2½ mon.	6 mon.	1½ years
Lateral incisor	4½ mon. in utero	Three fifths	3 mon.	7 mon.	1½ year
Cuspid	5 mon. in utero	One third	9 mon.	16 mon.	3¼ years
First molar	5 mon. in utero	Cusps united	5½ mon.	12 mon.	2½ years
Second molar	6 mon. in utero	Cusp tips still isolated	10 mon.	20 mon.	3 years

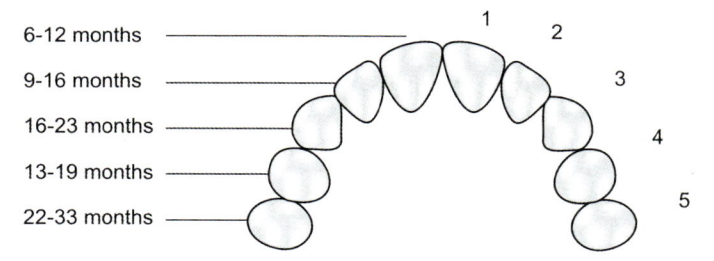

6-12 months —— 1

9-16 months —— 2

16-23 months —— 3

13-19 months —— 4

22-33 months —— 5

Fig. 18.11

MAXILLARY PRIMARY CENTRAL INCISOR

Labial Aspect

The labial surface is convex mesiodistally and less so incisocervically and is very smooth.

The incisal edge is nearly straight and is joined by the mesial and distal surface at an acute and at obtuse angle respectively.

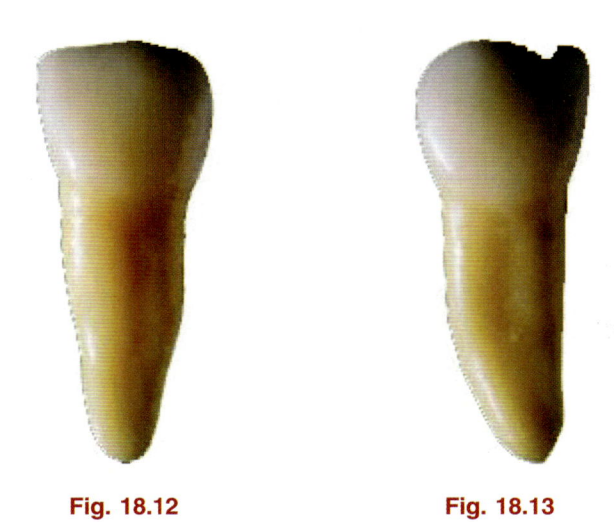

Fig. 18.12   Fig. 18.13

Lingual Aspect

The lingual surface presents a well defined angulum and marginal ridges. The depression between the marginal ridges and the angulum forms the lingual fossa.

Mesial and Distal Aspects

The mesial surface of the crown is slightly convex from the incisal edge to carnival third. The distal surface has a uniformly convex appearance from the vital edge to the cervical inclination of the incisal border.

196 Dental Anatomy

Root

The root is single and tapers to a blunt apex and exhibits a slight distal inclination. The mesial surface of the root usually exhibits a developmental groove.

DIFFERENCE BETWEEN MAXILLARY PRIMARY CENTRAL AND LATERAL INCISOR

The maxillary primary lateral incisor is similar to the central incisor from all aspects, but the crown is smaller in all aspects. Crown height is greater than mesio-distal width.

The root is long and flattened on mesial and distal surfaces.

MANDIBULAR PRIMARY CENTRAL INCISORS

This is the smallest tooth in human dentition.

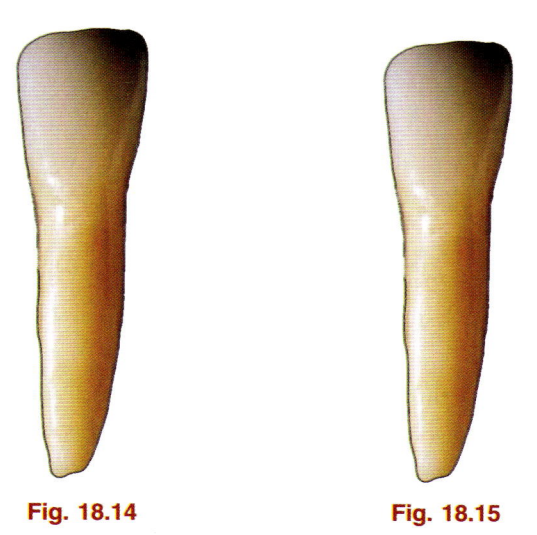

Fig. 18.14   Fig. 18.15

Labial Aspect

The labial surface is convex, smooth and symmetrical. The labial aspect is without development groove and angulum.

Lingual Aspect

The marginal ridges are not well defined and the lingual fossa is shallow. The angulum is well defined and occupies the cervical third of the lingual surface.

Mesial and Distal Aspects

They are triangular, smooth and convex. The mesioincisal angle is sharp and the distoincisal angle is rounded.

Root

The root is twice as long as the crown. It is cone shaped, slightly flattened on its mesial and distal aspects and tapers towards the apex.

DIFFERENCE BETWEEN PRIMARY MANDIBULAR CENTRAL AND LATERAL INCISOR

The deciduous incisors are smaller. The central incisor is somewhat larger in all dimensions except, labiolingually. The cervical margin is very prominent.

The root of the lateral incisor is slightly longer than the central. The angulum is very prominent and extends more incisally.

MAXILLARY PRIMARY CANINE

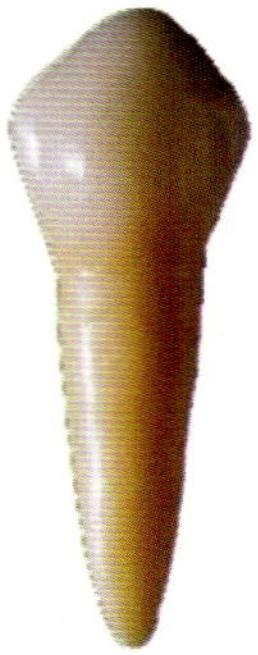

Fig. 18.16 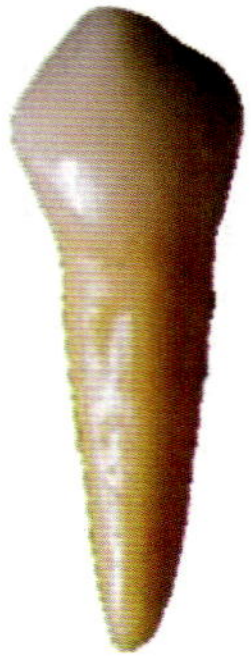   Fig. 18.17

Labial Aspect

The cervical ridge is prominent. The mesio incisal edge is longer than the distoincisal edge.

Lingual Aspect

It is mostly convex with a well-developed angulum and occupies half of the crown.

Mesial and Distal Aspect

They are convex and has a lingual tapering. The measurement labiolingual is greater.

Root

The root is long, thick in diameter is triangular in cross section and is tapering. The apex of the root is rounded.

DIFFERENCE BETWEEN PRIMARY MAXILLARY AND MANDIBULAR CANINE

The mandibular primary canine is not as bulbous labiolingually or as broad mesiodistally than the maxillary primary canine. The distoincisal edge is longer than the mesioincisal edge, this is opposite to maxillary primary canine.

The angulum is much smaller and occupies less than carnival third of the crown. The mesiodistal dimension is less and the cervico-incisal dimension is more when compared to the maxillary primary canine.

The root is proportionately larger and shows slight distal inclination near the applied end.

THE MAXILLARY PRIMARY FIRST MOLAR

The maxillary primary first molar is replaced by the first permanent premolar.

Fig. 18.18   Fig. 18.19

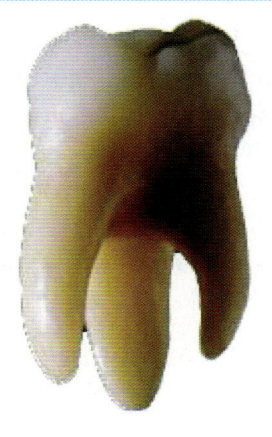

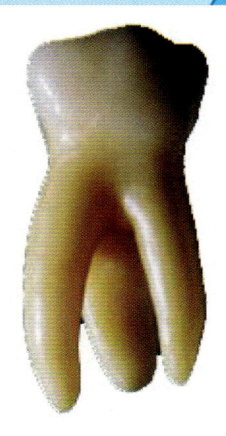

Buccal Aspect

This surface is convex in all directions. The mesiobuccal and disto-buccal cusps are viewed from this aspect. The cervical line is well-developed.

Lingual Aspect

Mesiolingual cusp forms the most of the occlusal border. Distolingual cusp is poorly defined.

Mesial Aspect

The mesial surface is greater in dimension at the cervical border than at the occlusal surface. The mesiolingual line angle is obtused.

Distal Aspect

The crown is narrower distally than mesially. The marginal ridge is fairly well developed.

Occlusal Aspect

The crown is broader on the buccal and mesial than the lingual and distal. The occlusal surface is made up of three cusps, i.e. mesiobuccal, distobuccal and the mesiolingual.

Roots

The roots are three in number, namely mesiobuccal, disto-buccal and lingual roots, and are divergent widely.

DIFFERENCE BETWEEN FIRST MAXILLARY PRIMARY MOLAR AND SECOND MAXILLARY PRIMARY MOLAR

The second primary molar is replaced by the permanent second premolar and are smaller in all dimensions than the first primary molar. It has four cusps, a central fissure, oblique ridge, a buccal and a lingual groove.

THE MANDIBULAR PRIMARY FIRST MOLAR

It is replaced by the first premolar in permanent dentition.

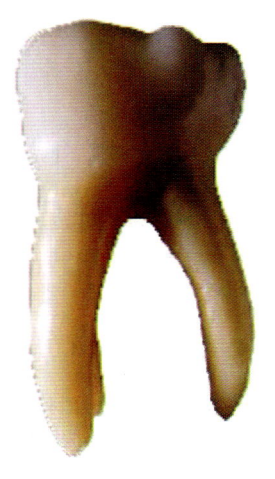

Fig. 18.20 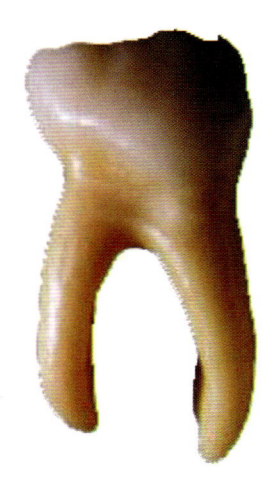   Fig. 18.21

Buccal Aspect

The crown is very wide mesiodistally and narrower buccolingually. The cervical line is sharp and larger mesiobuccal cusp and much smaller distobuccal cusp are seen.

Lingual Aspect

The lingual surface is convex mesio distally and cervicoocclusally. The mesiolingual cusp is larger, longer and sharper.

All three roots may be seen from this angle, but the distobuccal root is superimposed on the mesiobuccal root so that only the buccal surface and the apex of the latter may be seen. The point of bifurcation of the distobuccal root and the lingual root is near the cementoenamel junction as described heretofore as being typical.

Occlusal Aspect

The calibration of the distance between the mesiobuccal line angle and the distobuccal line angle is definitely greater than the calibration between the mesiolingual line angle and the distolingual line angle. Therefore, the crown outline converges lingually. Also, the calibration from the mesiobuccal line angle to the mesiolingual line angle is definitely greater than that found at the distal line angles. Therefore, the crown converges distally also. Nevertheless, these convergencies are not reflected entirely in the working occlusal surface because it is more nearly rectangular with the shortest sides of the rectangle represented by the marginal ridges. The occlusal surface is more nearly rectangular, with the shortest side of the rectangle represented by the marginal ridges.

The occlusal surface has a *central fossa*. There is a *mesial triangular fossa*, just inside the mesial marginal ridge, with a mesial pit in this fossa and a sulcus with its central groove connecting the two fossae. There is also a well-defined *buccal developmental groove* dividing the mesiobuccal cusp and the distobuccal cusp occlusally. There are:

Mesial Aspect

This surface is relatively flat mesiodistally and cervico-occlusally. The cervical line is convex towards the occlusal surface.

Distal Aspect

The distobuccal and distolingual cusps are nearly the same height. The cervical line is horizontal from buccal to lingual.

Occlusal Aspect

This surface is longer mesio-distally than bucco-lingually. The mesio-buccal, disto-buccal, mesiolingual and distolingual cusps are seen.

Roots

It has two roots a mesial and a distal, and is shorter than the permanent first molar. The mesial root is flat and distal root is rounded.

DIFFERENCE BETWEEN PRIMARY FIRST MANDIBULAR MOLAR AND MANDIBULAR SECOND MOLAR

This tooth is replaced by the second premolar in the permanent dentition.

They are smaller than the first mandibular molar. It has a strong large buccal cingulum and convex proximal surfaces. Mesiobuccal cusp, distobuccal cusp and the distal cusp are viewed from the buccal aspect. Occlusally it has a large central fossa and smaller mesial and distal triangular fossae.

There are two roots which are divergent like that in first deciduous molar and roots are extremely narrow mesiodistally and very broad buccolingually.

Introduction of Dentition

Table 18.2: Difference between deciduous and permanent dentitions

S.No.	Deciduous teeth	Permanent teeth
1.	The crown of primary teeth are wider mesiodistally	The crown is wider cervicoincisally
2.	The color is more whiter	The color is darker
3.	Less mineralized and is more opaque and whiter	It is more mineralized and it is translucent
4.	It has a prominent cervical marking	It has a less prominent cervical line
5.	Buccal and lingual aspects shows flat at cervical bulge	Buccal and lingual aspects shows greater degree at cervical bulge
6.	They have a marked cervical constriction	Permanent teeth will not have constricted cervical lines
7.	The primary teeth shows a greater degree of attrition due to less mineralization	Due to high mineralization the cusps show a greater variation
8.	The contact areas between primary molars are broader, flatter and situated farther gingivally	The contact areas are situated at the greater degree of convexity of the proximal surface of the tooth
9.	Deep pits and fissures are seen and more prone to dental caries	The pit and fissures are shallow and less prone to dental caries
10.	The inclination of enamel rods in the gingival one third of primary molars is towards the occlusal surface	The enamel rods in permanent teeth inclines horizontally
11.	Mamelons at the incisal edge of the anteriors are not seen	Mamelons at the incisal edge of the anteriors are present
12.	Overall the crown sizes of deciduous is smaller	Overall the crown size of permanent dentition is greater
13.	The cingulum is more prominent and extends more incisally	The cingulum is prominent but constraint to cervical 1/3rd
14.	The roots of primary teeth are longer and thinner.	The roots are at its standard size and uniformly thicker.

Contd[a]

204 Dental Anatomy

Contd[a]

S. No. Deciduous teeth	Permanent teeth
15. In primary molars the undivided part of the root area is much less extensive and the roots diverge widely and abrupthy from the short trunk	In permanent molars the undivided part of the root area is much more extensive and the roots diverge less wide and abrupt from the bigger trunk
16. The roots of primary teeth are more flared to allow for the development of the underlying permanent teeth	The roots in permanent teeth is not flared
17. The roots of primary teeth are fully formed about one year after eruption	It takes a longer duration
18. The roots of primary dentition undergo physiologic resorption	It tends to be pathologic.
19. The pulphorns are placed at higher level	The pulphorns follows the contour of the tooth.
20. There are no defined root canal entrance	There is a defined root canal entrance present

ABBREVIATIONS

BR	-	Buccal Root
BTR	-	Buccal Triangular Ridge
BC	-	Buccal Cusp
BCR	-	Buccal Cervical Ridge
BDG	-	Buccal Developmental Groove
C	-	Cingulum
CDG	-	Central Developmental Groove
CF	-	Central Fossa
CL	-	Cervical Line
DBC	-	Distobuccal Cusp
DBCR	-	Distobuccal Cusp Ridge
DBGD	-	Distobuccal Developmental Groove
DBR	-	Distobuccal Root
DC	-	Distal Cusp
DCA	-	Distal Contact Area

Introduction of Dentition

Table 18.3: Chronology of the human permanent dentition

Tooth	Hard tissue formation begins	Amount of enamel formed at birth	Enamel completed	Eruption	Root complete
Maxillary					
Central Incisor	3-4 months	—	4-5 years	7-8 years	10 years
Lateral incisor	10-12 months	—	4-5 years	8-9 years	11 years
Cuspid	4-5 months	—	6-7 years	11-12 years	13-15 years
First bicuspid	1½ - 1¾ years	—	5-6 years	10-11 years	12-13 years
Second bicuspid	2-2½ years	—	6-7 years	10-12 years	12-14 years
First molar	At birth	Sometimes a trace	2½-3 years	6-7 years	9-10 years
Second molar	2½-3 years	—	7-8 years	12-23 years	14-16 years
Mandibular					
Central incisor	3-4 months	—	4-5 years	6-7 years	9 years
Lateral incisor	3-4 months	—	4-5 years	7-8 years	10 years
Cuspid	4-5 months	—	6-7 years	9-10 years	12-14 years
First bicuspid	1¾ - 2 years	—	5-6 years	10-12 years	12-13 years
Second bicuspid	2¼-2½ years	—	6-7 years	11-12 years	13-14 years
First molar	At birth	Sometimes a trace	2½-3 years	6-7 years	9-10 years
Second molar	2½ - 3 years	—	7-8 years	11-13 years	14-15 years

206 Dental Anatomy

Table 18.4: Dimensions suggested for carving technique (Measurement table)

*In millimeters

Teeth	Cervico-incisal or occlusal length of crown	Length of root	Mesiodistal diameter of crown	Mesiodistal Diameter of crown at cervix	Labio or bucco lingual diameter of crown	Labio or bucco lingual diameter at cervix	Curvature of cervical line-mesial	Curvature of cervical line-distal
Maxillary central incisor	10.5*	13.0	8.5	7.0	7.0	6.0	3.5	2.5
Maxillary lateral incisor	9.0*	13.0	6.5	5.0	6.0	5.0	3.0	2.0
Maxillary canine	10.0	17.0	7.5	5.5	8.0	7.0	2.5	1.5
Maxillary 1st premolar	8.5	14.0	7.0	5.0	9.0	8.0	1.0	0.0
Maxillary 2nd premolar	8.5	14.0	7.0	5.0	9.0	8.0	1.0	0.0
Maxillary 1st molar	7.5	B L 12 13	10.0	8.0	11.0	10.0	1.0	0.0
Mandibular central incisor	9.0*	12.5	5.0	3.5	6.0	5.3	3.0	2.0
Mandibular lateral incisor	9.5*	14.0	5.5	4.0	6.5	5.8	3.0	2.0
Mandibular canine	11.0	16.0	7.0	5.5	7.5	7.0	2.5	1.0
Mandibular 1st premolar	8.5	14.0	7.0	5.0	7.5	6.5	1.0	0.0
Mandibular 2nd premolar	8.0	14.5	7.0	5.0	8.0	7.0	1.0	0.0
Mandibuar 1st molar	7.5	14.0	11.0	9.0	10.5	9.0	1.0	0.0

Introduction of Dentition   207

DCR	-	Distal Cusp Ridge
DLC	-	Distolingual Cusp
DLCR	-	Distolingual Cusp Ridge
DLF	-	Distolingual Fossa
DMR	-	Distal Marginal Ridge
DR	-	Distal Root
DTF	-	Distal Triangular Fossa
FC	-	Fifth cusp
IR	-	Incisal Ridge
LC	-	Lingual Cusp
LDG	-	Lingual Developmental Groove
LF	-	Lingual Fossa
LIE	-	Labioincisal Edge
LIE	-	Linguoincisal Edge
LR	-	Lingual Ridge
LR	-	Lingual Root
MBC	-	Mesiobuccal Cusp
MBCR	-	Mesiobuccal Cusp Ridge
MBR	-	Mesiobuccal Root
MCA	-	Mesial Contact Area
MCR	-	Mesial Cusp Ridge
MDD	-	Mesial Development Depression
MLC	-	Mesiolingual Cusp
MLCR	-	Mesiolingual Cusp Ridge
MLDG	-	Mesiolingual Developmental Groove
MLF	-	Mesiolingual Fossa
MMDG	-	Mesial Marginal Developmental Groove
MMR	-	Mesial Marginal Ridge
MR	-	Mesial Root
MTF	-	Mesial Triangular Fossa
OR	-	Oblique Ridge
SG	-	Supplementary Groove

Fig. 18.22   Fig. 18.23

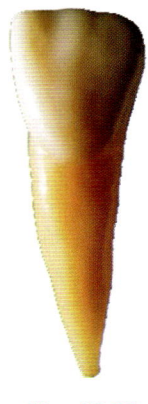

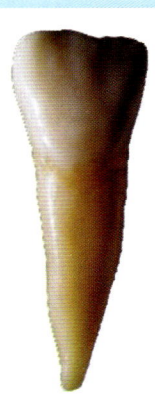

MAXILLARY CENTRAL INCISOR

Introduction

- The maxillary central incisor is the wider mesiodistally.
- The labial face is less convex than the maxillary lateral incisor or canine, which gives the central incisor a squared or rectangular appearance.
- The mesial incisal angle is relatively sharp, the distal incisal angle rounded.
- The labial surface or the crown is usually convex.
- When the tooth is newly erupted, mamelons will be seen.
- Lingual area is concave.

Labial Aspect

- The crown of the average central incisor will be 10 to 11 mm long from the highest point on the cervical line to the lowest point on the incisal edge.
- The mesiodistal measurement will be 8-9 mm wide at the contact areas.
- The distal outline of the crown is more convex than the mesial outline.
- The distoincisal angle is not so sharp as the mesioincisal angle.

- The incisal outline is usually regular and straight in a mesiodistal dissection after the tooth has been in function long enough to obliterate the mamelons.
- The cervical outline is towards root wise.
- The root of the central incisor from the labial aspect is cone-shaped with blunt apex.

Lingual Aspect

- This aspect has convexities and a concavity.
- Below the cervical line a smooth convexity is found and is called as cingulum.
- Mesially and distally confluent with the cingulum are the marginal ridges.
- Between the marginal ridges, below the cingulum, a shallow concavity is present called the lingual fossa.
- Usually these are developmental grooves extending from the cingulum into the lingual fossae.
- The crown and root taper lingually.

Mesial Aspect

- The crown is wedge-shaped.
- Labio-lingual bulk at cervical shows a great degree from this aspect.
- Usually a line drawn through the crown and the root from the mesial aspect through the center of the tooth will bisect the apex of the root and also the incisal ridge of the crown.
- The labial outline of the crown from the crest of curvature to the incisal ridge is very slightly convex.
- The cervical line outlining the cementoenamel junction mesially on the maxillary central incisor curves incisally to a noticeable degree.
- The root of this tooth from this aspect is cone shaped, and the apex of the root is usually bluntly rounded.

Distal Aspect

- When looking at the central incisor from this aspect, we may note that the crown gives impression of being somewhat thicker toward the incisal third.
- The curvature of the cervical line is toward crown and is less in extent on the distal than on the mesial surface

Incisal Aspect

- From this aspect, the labial face of the crown is relatively broad and flat in comparison with the lingual surface.
- The cervical portion of the crown labially is convex.
- The incisal ridge may be seen clearly.
- The outline of the lingual portion tapers lingually towards the cingulum.
- The mesial and distal marginal ridges are seen from this aspect.

DIFFERENCES BETWEEN CENTRAL AND LATERAL PERMANENT MAXILLARY INCISORS

Labial Aspect

It has a more rounded incisal/wide and rounded incisal angle mesially and distally.

The crown is smaller in all dimensions when compared with central incisor.

The mesioincisal angle and distoincisal angle of outline is more rounded habit surface is more convex than central incisor. Narrow mesiodistally and shorter cervicoincisally when compared with central incisor.

Lingual Aspect

The lingual fossa is more concave. It tapers towards lingually.

Mesial Aspect

Mesially the heavy development of the incisal ridge accordingly makes the incisal portion appear somewhat thicker than that of center incisor.

Distal Aspect

The width of the crown distally appears thicker than it does on the mesial aspect from marginal ridge to labial face.

Incisal Aspect

Labiolingual dimension may be greater than usual in comparison with the mesiodistal dimension.

All the maxillary lateral incisors exhibit more convexity labially and lingually from the incisal aspect than maxillary central incisors.

PERMANENT MANDIBULAR INCISORS

Introduction

1. The mandibular incisors are four in number.
2. The mandibular central incisors are centered in the mandible, one on either side of the median line, with the mesial surface of each one in contact with the mesial surface of the other.
3. The right and left mandibular lateral or second incisors are distal to the central incisors.
4. They are in contact with central incisors mesially and with the canines distally.
5. Normally the mandibular central incisor is the smallest tooth in the dental arches.

MANDIBULAR CENTRAL INCISOR

Labial Aspect

1. The mesial and distal sides of the crown taper evenly from the contact areas to the narrow cervix.

Fig. 18.24 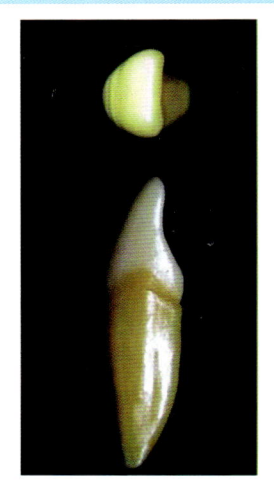   Fig. 18.25

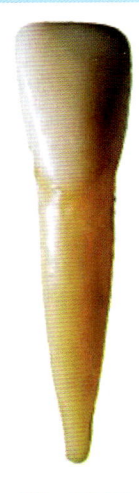

2. The mesial and distal root outlines are straight with the mesial and distal outlines of the crown down to the apical portion.
3. The cervical line is pointed towards the roots.
4. The apical third of the root terminates in a small pointed taper, in most cases curving distally, sometimes the roots are straight.
5. The labial face of mandibular central incisor crown is ordinarily smooth with a flattened surface at the incisal third, the middle third is more convex, narrowing down to the convexity of the root at the cervical portion.

Lingual Aspect

1. The lingual surface of the crown is smooth, with very slight concavity.
2. The marginal ridges are more prominent near the incisal edges.
3. This aspect shows MMR, DMR, Lingual/Fossa, Incisal Ridge, Cingulum.

4. The cingulum is present on the lingual surface just above the cervical line.
5. The cervical lines is pointed towards root surface.

Mesial Aspect

1. The curvature labially and lingually above the cervical line is less than that found on maxillary incisors.
2. The curvature of the cervical line representing the cementoenamel junction on the mesial surface is marked, curving incisally approximately one third the length of the crown.
3. The root outlines from the mesial aspect are straight with the crown outline from the cervical line.
4. The mesial surface of the crown is convex and smooth at the incisal third and becomes broader and flatter.
5. The mesial surface of the root is flat labio-lingually just below the cervical line.
6. Most of these roots have a broader developmental depression for the most of the root length.

Distal Aspect

1. The cervical line facing the crown surface is less of 1 mm to that of mesial aspect.
2. The development depression on the distal surface of the root may be more marked with a deeper and more well-defined developmental groove at its center.

Incisal Aspect

1. This aspect illustrates the bilateral symmetry of the mandibular central incisor.
2. The incisal edge is almost at right angles to a line bisecting the crown labio-lingually.
3. They serve as a mark of identification in differentiation between mandibular central and lateral incisors.

4. The labial surface of the crown is wider mesiodistally than the lingual surface.
5. The other reactors, like MMR, DMR, incisal ridge cingulum are seen.

MANDIBULAR LATERAL INCISOR

1. The mandibular lateral incisor is the second mandibular tooth from the median line, right or left.
2. The mandibular central incisor and mandibular lateral incisor operate in the dental arch as a team, their functional form is related.

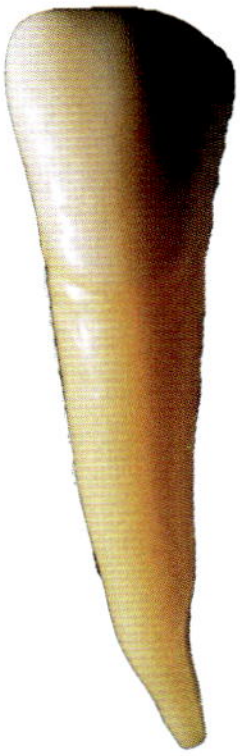

Fig. 18.26

Labial and Lingual Aspect

The labial and lingual aspects show the added fraction of approximately 1 mm of crown diameter mesiodistally added to the distal half.

Mesial and Distal Aspect

1. The mesial side of the crown is often longer than distal side, causing the incisal ridge, which is straight to slope downwards in a distal direction.

2. The distal contact area is more towards the cervical than the mesial contact area to contact properly the mesial contact area of the mandibular canine.
3. The crown of the mandibular lateral incisor is somewhat longer than that of central incisor. The tooth is, therefore a little larger in all dimensions.

Incisal Aspect

1. The incisal aspect of the mandibular lateral incisor provides a feature that can usually serve to identify this tooth.
2. The incisal edge is not at an approximate right angle to a line bisecting the crown, and root labio-lingually as in central incisor.
3. The edge follows the curvature of the mandibular dental arch, giving the crown of the mandibular lateral incisor the appearance of being twisted slightly on its root base.
4. The other common features like, lingual fossa, MMR, DMR, cingulum, incisal ridges are seen from this aspect.

MAXILLARY AND MANDIBULAR CANINE

Introduction

1. The maxillary and mandibular canine bear a close resemblance to each other and their functions are closely related.

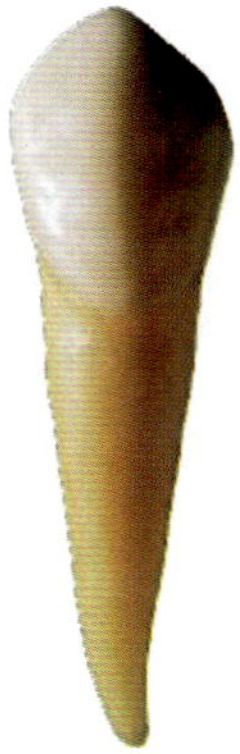

Fig. 18.27

2. They are the longer teeth in the mouth.
3. They are also called "corner stone" in dental arch.

Labial Aspect

1. From the labial view, the mesial half of the crown resembles a portion of an incisor, whereas the distal half resembles as portion of a premolar.
2. The mesial contact with the lateral incisor and distal with the first premolar.
3. The labial surface shows convexity.
4. The cervical line labially is convex towards root portion.
5. This surface has got three labial lobes, the middle labial lobe is very prominent and thus forms a cusp.
6. The cusps has the mesial cusp ridge slope and distal cusp ridge slope, the mesial cusp ridge slope is shorter than the distal cusp ridge slope.
7. The root appears conically in for with a bluntly pointed apex.
8. The labial surface of the root is smooth, convex, distally pointed.

Lingual Aspect

1. The cingulum is large-well prominent and in some instances is pointed like a small cusps.
2. The cervical line is pointed towards the root surface.
3. Mesial marginal ridges and distal marginal ridge extends towards cingulum.
4. This ridges forms a concavity and represents mesial and distal lingual fossae.
5. The lingual portion is narrower than the labial portion.
6. The other landmarks from this aspect are, prominent cingulum, M&F, D&F, MMR, DMR, Lingual ridge, MCR, DCR.

Mesial Aspect

1. The mesial aspect resembles functional form of anterior tooth.
2. The outline of the crown is wedge-shaped and measurement is greater in the cervical third.

Introduction of Dentition 217

3. The entire labial outline from the mesial aspect exhibits more convexity.
4. The cervical line is pointed towards a cusp.
5. The outline of the root is conical with a tapered or bluntly pointed apex, with a greater in dimension labiolingually.
6. The mesial surface of the root appears broad with a shallow development depressions.

Distal Aspect

The distal aspect is similar to the mesial aspect and differs from that as follows:
1. The cervical line exhibits less curvature towards the cusps.
2. The distal marginal ridge is heavier.
3. The developmental depressions are more prominent.

Incisal Aspect

1. The laibo-lingual dimension is greater than the mesio-distal.
2. The ridge of the middle labial lobe is very noticeable labially from this aspect.
3. The cingulum development makes up the cervical third of the crown lingually.
4. The line bisecting the cusps and cusps ridges drawn in the mesiodistal direction is almost always straight and bisects the short arcs representative of the mesial and distal contact areas.
5. The other features like MCR, DCR, slope, cingulum lingual ridge, MLF, DLF seen from this aspect.

MANDIBULAR CANINE

1. The maxillary and mandibular canine bears close resemblances except the following differences:
2. The mandibular canine will have a bifurcated root.

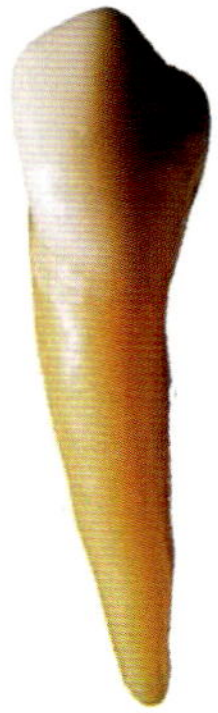

Fig. 18.28

Labial Aspect

1. The meisodistal dimension is less.
2. The cervical incisal length of the crown is more by 1 mm.

Lingual Aspect

1. The lingual aspect is more flatter and cingulum is poorly developed.
2. The mesial and distal marginal ridges are less prominent.

Mesial Aspect

1. The cervical line curves more towards incisor portion.
2. The cingulum is not prominent. The developmental depressions are seen from this aspect.

Distal Aspect

Developmental depressions are seen and the root apex is more pointed.

Incisal Aspect

1. The mesio-distal dimension of mandibular canine is less than the labio-lingual dimension.
2. The cusp tip and mesial cusp ridge are more inclined lingually.

THE PERMANENT MAXILLARY PREMOLAR

Introduction

1. The maxillary premolars are four in number—two in right maxilla and two in left maxilla.
2. They are also called as bicuspid.
3. Premolars are those teeth that succeeds the deciduous molars.
4. It has buccal and lingual cusps.
5. The buccal cusp is usually 1 mm longer than lingual cusp.

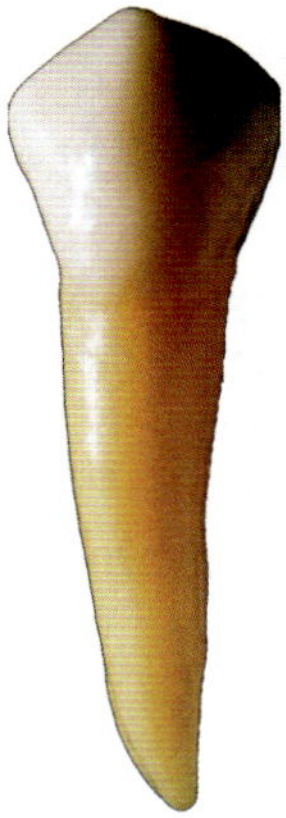

Fig. 18.29 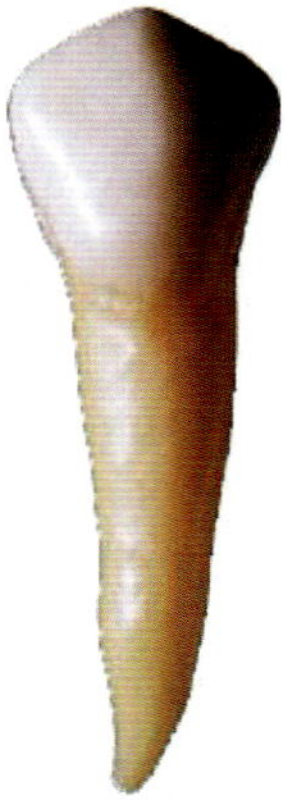 Fig. 18.30

Buccal Aspect

1. The crown is roughly trapezoidal.
2. The crown exhibits little curvature at the cervical line.
3. The mesial slope of the buccal cusp is rather straight and longer than the distal slope.
4. The distal contact area is represented by a broader curvature than is found mesially.
5. The continuous ridge from cusp tip to cervical margin on the buccal surface of the crown is called the buccal ridge.
6. The middle buccal lobe, the mesio and distobuccal lobes are the three lobes seen.
7. The roots are 3 or 4 mm shorter than those of the maxillary canine.

Lingual Aspect

1. The crown tapers towards the lingual, since the lingual cusp is narrower mesiodistally than the buccal cusp.
2. The crown is convex at all points.
3. The smooth lingual portion that terminates at the point of the lingual cusp is called the lingual ridge.

4. The mesial and distal outlines of the lingual portion of the crown are convex.
5. The cervical line lingually is regular, with slight curvature towards the root.
6. The lingual portion of the crown is narrower than the buccal portion, so it is possible to see part of mesial and distal buccal surfaces of crown and root from this aspect.
7. Roots are smooth and convex at all points.
8. The lingual root is more blunt than the buccal root apex.

Mesial Aspect

1. Two roots, one buccal and one lingual are clearly outlined from mesial aspect.
2. The cervical line may be regular in outline, towards the crown surface.
3. From the mesial aspect, the buccal outline of the crown curves outwards below the cervical line.
4. The buccal outline continues as a line of less convexity to the tip of the buccal cusp.
5. The lingual cusp is always shorter than the buccal cusp, the average difference being about 1 mm
6. A deep developmental depression is seen between the roots and ends at the root bifurcation.
7. A well-defined developmental groove in the enamel of the mesial marginal ridge is seen.
8. The buccal root shows lingual inclination.

MAXILLARY SECOND PREMOLAR

Difference between first and second premolars are:

Buccal Aspect

1. The crown is buccally smaller, cervico-occlusally and mesiodistally.
2. Usually the root length is greater.

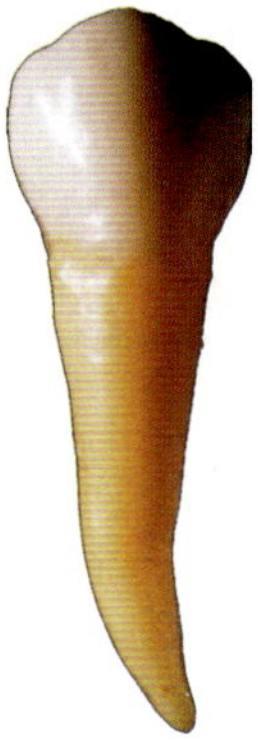

Fig. 18.31   Fig. 18.32

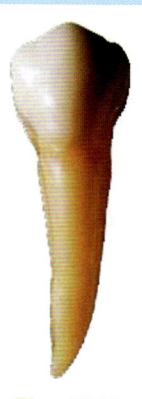

3. Mesial cusp ridge slope is shorter than the distal cusp ridge slope (opposite of first premolar) but same as canine.
4. Buccal ridge is not so prominent.

Lingual Aspect

1. The lingual cusp is longer, making the crown longer on the lingual side.

Mesial Aspect

1. The cusps of the second premolar are shorter.
2. There is no deep developmental depression on the mesial surface of the crown as on the first premolar.
3. There is no deep developmental groove crossing the mesial marginal ridge.

Distal Aspect

1. There is no outstanding variations to be noted when viewed from the distal aspect.

Occlusal Aspect

1. The central developmental groove is shorter and more irregular.

2. The outline of the crown is more rounded or oval.
3. There are supplementary grooves radiating from the central groove.

THE PERMANENT MANDIBULAR PREMOLARS

Introduction

- The mandibular premolars are four in number.
- Two are situated in the right side of the mandible and two in the left side.
- They are immediately posterior to mandibular canines and anterior to the molars.
- They are developed from four lobes, as were the maxillary premolars.
- The first premolar has large buccal cusps, which is long and well formed, with a small non-functioning lingual cusp.
- The second premolar has three well formed cusps in most cases, on large buccal cusp and two smaller lingual cusps.
- The form of both mandibular premolars fails to conform to the implications of the term "Bicuspid". The term implying two functioning cusps.
- The first premolar is always smaller than the second mandibular premolar.
- The mandibular second premolar has more of the characteristics of a small molar because its lingual cusps are well-developed.

MANDIBULAR FIRST PREMOLAR

It is the fourth tooth from the median line and the first posterior tooth in the mandible.

The characteristics that resemble those of the mandibular canine are as follows:
- The buccal cusp is long and sharp and is only occluding cusp.
- The buccolingual measurement is similar to that of the canine.

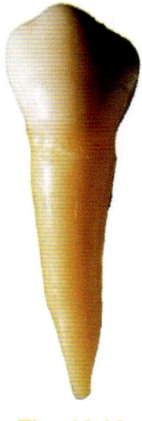

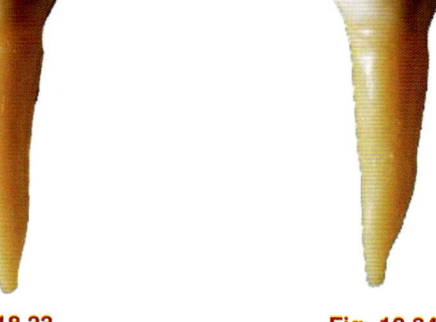

Fig. 18.33   Fig. 18.34

- The occlusal surface slopes sharply lingually in cervical direction.
- The mesiobuccal cusp ridge is shorter than the distobuccal cusp ridge.

The outline form of the occlusal aspect resembles the outline form of the incisal aspect of the canine.

Buccal Aspect

1. The middle buccal lobe is well developed resulting in a large, pointed buccal cusp.
2. The mesial cusp ridges slope shorter than the distal cusp ridge slope.
3. From the buccal aspect, the crown is roughly trapezoidal.
4. The mesial and distal slope of the buccal cusp usually shows some concavity.
5. The tip of the buccal cusp is pointed.
6. The distal slope of the buccal cusp usually exhibits some concavity.
7. The root of this tooth is 3 or 4 mm shorter than that of the mandibular canine.

8. The continuous ridge from the cervical margin to the cusp tip is called the buccal ridge.
9. The buccal surface of the crown is more convex.

Lingual Aspect

- The crown of the mandibular first premolar tapers towards the lingual since the lingual measurement mesiodistally is less than that buccally.
- The lingual cusp is always small.
- The major portion of the crown is made up of the middle buccal lobe.
- The crown and the root tapers markedly towards the lingual, so that most of the mesial and distal surfaces of both may be seen from the lingual aspect.
- The occlusal surface slopes greatly toward the lingual in a cervical direction down to the short lingual cusp.
- Most of the occlusal surface of this tooth can be seen from this aspect.
- The cervical portion of the crown lingually is narrow and convex.
- Although the lingual cusp is short and poorly developed, it shows a pointed tip.
- The mesial and distal occlusal fossae are on each side of the triangular ridge.
- A characteristic of the lingual surface is the mesiolingual developmental groove, which acts as a line of demarcation between the mesiobuccal lobe and the lingual lobe.

Mesial Aspect

- The surface of the crown presents an overhang above the root trunk in a lingual direction.
- The tip of the cusp will be on a line approximately with the lingual border of the root.

Introduction of Dentition 225

- When viewed from the medial aspect of ten shows the buccal cusp centered over the root.
- The buccal outline of the crown from this aspect is prominently curved from the cervical line to the tip of the buccal cusp.
- The lingual outline of the crown is less convex than that of the buccal surface.
- The mesiobuccal lobe development is prominent from this aspect, is created by its form the mesial contact area and the mesial marginal ridge.
- The cervical line on the mesial surface is rather regular, curving occlusally.
- The root outline from this aspect is tapered from the cervix.
- The lingual outline may be straight, the buccal outline more curved.

Distal Aspect

- The major portion of this surface of the crown is smoothly convex, the distal contact area is broader than the mesial.
- The distal contact area is broader than the mesial.
- The curvature of the cervical line distally is towards crown surface.
- The surface of the root distally exhibits more convexity than was found mesially.
- A shallow development depression is centered on the root.

Occlusal Aspect

- The usual outline from this aspect is roughly diamond-shaped and in circular form.
- The middle buccal lobe makes up the major bulk of the tooth crown.
- The buccal ridge is prominent.
- The marginal ridges are well developed.
- The lingual cusp is small.
- The occlusal surface shows a heavy buccal triangular ridge and small buccal triangular ridge.

- The occlusal surface harbors two depressions namely mesial and distal fossae.
- The most common type of mandibular first premolar shows a mesiolingual developmental depression and groove.

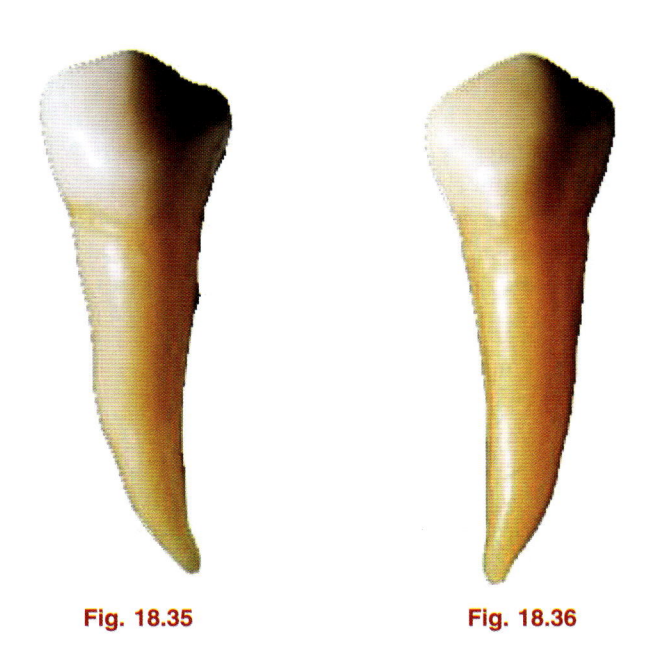

Fig. 18.35   Fig. 18.36

MANDIBULAR SECOND PREMOLAR

The single root of the second premolar is larger and longer than that of first premolar.

Buccal Aspect

From this aspect, the mandibular second premolar presents a shorter buccal cusp than the first premolar.

Lingual Aspect

The lingual lobes are developed to a greater degree.

Mesial Aspect

- The crown and the root are wider buccolingually.
- There is no mesiolingual developmental groove on the crown portion, the apex of the roots is usually more blunt on the second premolar.

Distal Aspect

In this aspect more of the occlusal surface may be seen, this is possible since the distal marginal ridge is at a lower level than the mesial marginal ridge when we pose the tooth vertically.

Occlusal Aspect

The mesial developmental groove travels in a mesiobuccal direction and ends in the mesial triangular fossae just distal to the mesial marginal ridge.

The distal development groove travels in a distobuccal direction, somewhat shorter than the mesial groove and ends in the distal triangular fossae, mesial to the distal marginal ridge.

MAXILLARY MOLARS

Introduction

1. These tooth assist the mandibular molars in performing the major portion of work in mastication of food.
2. They are largest and strongest maxillary teeth, because of their bulkness.
3. Their dimensions are greater in every aspect.
4. The root portion may be not longer than the premolars.
5. They have 3 roots—2 buccal and 1 palatal.
6. The first molar appears in oral cavity when at age of 6 years.

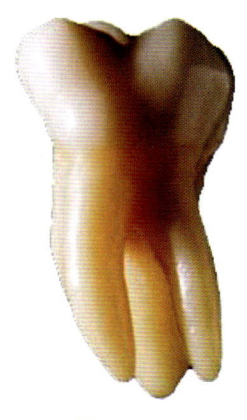

228 Dental Anatomy

Fig. 18.37 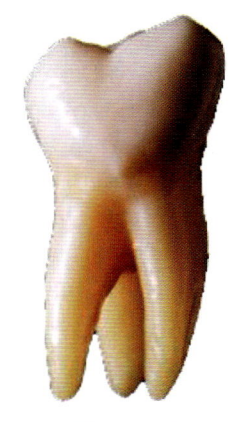 **Fig. 18.38**

7. The first molar erupts posterior to second deciduous molar, therefore it is not a succeedaneous tooth because it has no predecessor.

FIRST MAXILLARY MOLARS

Introduction

- The crown of this tooth is wider buccolingually than mesiodistally.
- Extradimension buccolingually is about 1 mm.
- First molar is normally largest tooth in maxillary arch.
- Four well developed cusps—mesiobuccal, distobuccal, mesiolingual distolingual.
- Additional cusp or supplementary cusp of carabelli is present.
- It is found lingual to mesiolingual cusp.
- Mesiolingual cusp is largest.
- The 5th cusp helps in identifying the first molar.
- Three roots mesiobuccal, distobuccal and palatal roots are present.
- Mesiobuccal root is not as long but is broader buccolingually.
- Distobuccal root is the smallest of three.

Buccal Aspect

1. The crown is roughly trapezoidal with cervical and occlusal outlines representing the uneven sides.
2. The cervical is shorter on the uneven sides.
3. The mesiobuccal cusp is broader than the distobuccal cusp.
4. The mesial slope meets the distal slope at an obtuse angle.
5. The mesial slope of distobuccal cusp meets the distal slope at 90 degree angle.
6. The buccal developmental groove divides the two buccal cusps.
7. The cervical line of crown does not have much curvature from mesial to distal. However, it is not as smooth and regular with that found on other teeth, the line is generally convex towards the root.
8. All the three roots may be seen from buccal aspect.
9. The mesial buccal root curves distally starting at middle third.
10. The distal root is straighten.
11. The point of bifurcation of two buccal roots is located 4 mm above the cervical line.
12. Molar roots originate as a single root on base or crown.
13. The common root base is called root trunk.

Lingual Aspect or Palatal Aspect

1. The distolingual cusp is rounded, spheroidal and smooth.
2. The lingual cusps are the only one to be seen from lingual aspect.
3. The lingual developmental groove starts in center of lingual surface mesiodistally, curves sharply to distal surface as it crosses between the cusps and continues on occlusal surface.
4. The 5th cusp appears attached to mesiolingual surface of mesiolingual cusp.
5. All 3 roots are visible from this aspect.
6. The palatal root is conical, terminating in bluntly rounded apex.

7. All the mesial outlines of mesio-buccal root may be seen and part of its apex.
8. The distal outline of distobuccal root is seen above its middle third including all its apical outline.

Mesial Aspect

1. The mesiobuccal root hides the distobuccal root.
2. The mesiobuccal root is broad and flattened on its mesial surface.
3. The width of mesiobuccal root near the crown from buccal surface to the point of bifcuration on root trunk is 2/3rd of crown mesurement buccolingually at cervical line.
4. Although the palatal root is rounded the root appears more pointed towards the end than the mesiobuccal root.

Distal Aspect

1. The distal surface of the crown is generally convex with smoothly rounded surface except for a small area near the distobuccal root at cervical third.
2. This concavity continues on the distal surface of distobuccal root, from cervical line to the area of root that is on a level with bifurcation separation the disto-buccal and lingual roots.
3. The distobuccal root is narrower at its base than either of others.
4. The bifurcation here is more apical than either of other two areas of the tooth.

Occlusal Aspect

1. It is rhomboidal in shape.
2. *Cusps:*
    i. Mesiolingual cusp largest
    ii. Mesiobuccal
    iii. Distolingual
    iv. Distobuccal
    v. Cusp of Carabelli

3. Developmentally only three major cusps: Mesiolingual, mesiobuccal and distobuccal called maxillary molar primary cusp triangle.
4. The distolingual cusp progressively becomes smaller and 2nd and 3rd molars often disappearing.
5. Two major fossae—two minor fossae.
6. Major fossae—central fossa, distal fossa.
7. Central fossa is present mesial to oblique ridge and is triangular in shape.
8. Distal fossa is linear and placed distal to oblique ridge.
9. Oblique ridge runs between mesio-lingual and distobuccal cusps.
10. Minor fossae—mesial triangular fossa is present distal to mesial marginal ridge, distal triangular fossa present mesial to distal marginal ridge.

Oblique ridge, crossed occlusal surface obliquely the union of triangular ridges of distobuccal cusp and distal ridge of cusps forms its oblique ridge.

DIFFERENCE BETWEEN MAXILLARY FIRST MOLAR AND MAXILLARY SECOND MOLAR

The maxillary second molar supplements the first molar in function.

Buccal Aspect

The crown is little shorter cervico-occlusally and narrower mesiodistally than the maxillary first molar. The distobuccal cusp is smaller.

The apex of the mesiobuccal root is on a line with the buccal groove of the crown instead of the tip of the mesiobuccal cusp, as we found on the first molar.

Lingual Aspect

- The distolingual cusp of the crown is smaller.
- The fifth cusp or cusp of Carabelli is absent.

232 Dental Anatomy

Mesial Aspect

The buccolingual dimension is about the same as that of the first molar, but the crown length is less.

Distal Aspect

Because the distobuccal cusp is smaller than in the maxillary first molar, more of the mesiobuccal cusp may be seen from this angle.

Occlusal Aspect

The mesiobuccal and mesiolingual cusps are just as large and well developed as in the first molar, but the distobuccal and distolingual cusp are smaller and less well developed.

MAXILLARY THIRD MOLAR

Most of the maxillary third molars are well developed as the second molar. They are also called as wise done tooth and also called as non-functional teeth. The most of the roots are fused in third molar. The distobuccal cusps will be disintegrated especially in maxillary second and third molars.

MANDIBULAR FIRST MOLAR

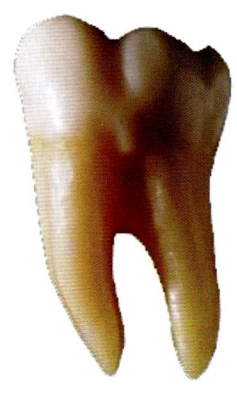

Fig. 18.39

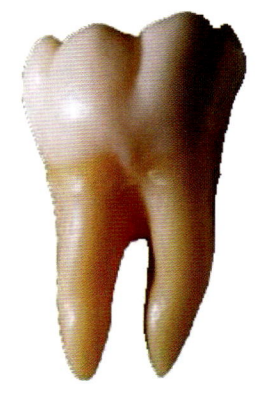

Fig. 18.40

Introduction

1. Mandibular molar is the largest tooth in the mandibular arch.
2. It has five well-developed cusps. Two buccal, two lingual and one distal cusps.
3. Two well-developed roots, one mesial, one distal which are broad buccolingually.
4. The root always curves distally in respect of their quadrant.

CHRONOLOGY OF MANDIBULAR FIRST MOLAR

First evidence of calcification - At birth
Crown completed   - 2½ – 3 years
Eruption   - 6 – 7 years
Root completed   - 9 – 10 years

Buccal Aspect

1. It is roughly trapezoidal in shape.
2. All the five cusps are viewed from this aspect.
3. The lingual cusps are seen from this aspect, because they are placed at the higher level.
4. Mesiobuccal and distobuccal developmental grooves are seen.
5. Buccal cusps are relatively flat.
6. *Cervical line:* Commonly regular in outline and dipping apically towards root bifurcation.
7. *Root:* The distal root is less curved than the mesial root.
8. Considerable variations are seen in the length of the root, i.e. mesial and distal.
9. The point of bifurcation of root is situated at 3 mm at the cervical line.
10. Developmental depressions are seen in their root trunk.

Lingual Aspect

1. Three cups will be seen, two lingual *lingual portion* of the distal cusps.

2. The two lingual cusps ridge are pointed well so that buccal cusps are not viewed from this aspect.
3. The mesial-lingual cusp is wider than the distolingual cusps.
4. The lingual developmental groove seen as a line of demarcation between lingual cusps.
5. The mesial aspect from this view will be convex from the cervical line.
6. The cervical line is towards the root bifurcation.
7. The contact point is higher in mesial than the distal.
8. The root bifucation starts 4 mm below the cervical line.

Mesial Aspect

1. Mesiobuccal and mesiolingual cusps and mesial root is viewed.
2. The buccolingual portion at the mesial side is greater than the buccolingual portion of the distal side.
3. The mesial root is broader than the distal root, that is buccolingually.
4. Since the mesial portion of the tooth are broader and the mesial cusps are higher, the distal portion of the tooth cannot be seen from this angle.
5. In comparison to that of second mandibular premolar all the aspects show similar in less mm.
6. Buccal aspect shows convexity.
7. The cervical line is towards the surface of the tooth or crown.
8. The mesial surface of the mesial root is convex at the buccal and the lingual borders.

Distal Aspect

1. The outline of the distal aspect is similar to that of mesial aspect.
2. Since the buccolingual diameter is seen less, the occlusal surface are viewed more in this aspect.
3. The distal portion of the crown is convex.

Introduction of Dentition 235

4. The distal contact area appearing at its distal contour.
5. The cervical line distally will be seen towards crown surface.
6. The end of the distobuccal developmental groove is seen in this aspect.
7. Developmental depressions are seen on the distal root.
8. The lingual border of the mesial root is seen from this aspect.
9. The distal root is narrower buccolingually than mesial root.

Occlusal Aspect

1. It looks hexagonal from the occlusal aspect.
2. The crown measurement is 1 mm more greater mesiodistally than the buccolingually.
3. The mesiobuccal cusps are less larger than the lingual cusps.
4. The distal cusps are smaller.
5. One major fossa, two minor fossae is seen.
6. The major fossa is the central fossa placed between the buccal and lingual cusp ridge.
7. Two minor fossae:
   1. Mesial triangular fossa
   2. Distal triangular fossa.
8. Mesial triangular fossa placed immediately distal to mesial marginal ridges.
9. Distal triangular fossa placed immediately mesial to distal marginal ridges.
10. The developmental grooves of both, passing the mesial and distal triangular fossae of the lingual and buccal aspects, always, starts from the central pit of the central fossa.

DIFFERENCE BETWEEN MANDIBULAR FIRST AND SECOND MOLAR

Mandibular second molar supplements the first molar in functions. The crown has four well developed cusps—two buccal and two lingual. There is no fifth distal cusp. The tooth has two well developed mesial and distal roots.

Buccal Aspect

Mesiobuccal and disto buccal cusps are viewed from this aspect.

The crown is shorter cervico-occlusally and narrow mesiodistally than in the first molar. The roots may be shorter, closer and fused type.

Lingual Aspect

The crown and root converge lingually but to slight degree. The cervical line shows less curvature being straight and regular in outline buccolingually.

Distal Aspect

From the distal aspect the second molar is similar in form to the first molar except for the absence of a distal cusp and a distobuccal grooves.

Occlusal Aspect

Small cusp of distal cusps are absent. Many of them are rectangular from the occlusal aspect. Most second molars exhibit more curvature of the outline of the crown distally than mesially.

MANDIBULAR THIRD MOLAR

The mandibular third molar is also called as wisdom teeth. It is a non-functioning teeth. Most of the third molars will be in impacted condition. The aspects will be generally resembling to that of the first molar. The crown is wide at the contact point. It usually have the same four cusps as the second molar and mesial and distal roots which may be fused. The occlusal surface more or less looks round in shape.

DENTAL OCCLUSION

Angle defined occlusion as the normal relation of the occlusal inclined planes of the teeth when the jaws are closed.

Introduction of Dentition 237

Terms Used in Studying Occlusion

- Ideal occlusion
- Physiologic occlusion
- Balanced occlusion
- Functional occlusion
- Therapeutic occlusion
- Traumatic occlusion
- Trauma from occlusion

Periods of Occlusal Development

1. Pre-dental period
2. Deciduous dentition period.   First transitional period
3. The mixed dentition period   Inter transitional period
4. The permanent dentition period.   Second transitional period

Types of Cusps

- Centric holding cusps.
- Non-supporting cusps.

Arrangements of Teeth in Humans

a. *Cusp-Fossa Occlusion:* In this type of occlusion, the stamp cusp at one teeth occludes in a single fossa of a single opponent.

b. *Cusp-Embrasure Occlusion:* In this type of arrangement, each tooth occludes with two opposing teeth.

Imaginary Occlusal Planes and Curves

The imaginary occlusal planes and curves are:
1. Curve of Spee
2. Curve of Wilson
3. Curve of Monson

Curve of Spee

It refers to the antero-posterior curvature of the occlusal surface beginning from the tip of the lower cuspid and following the cusp tips of the bicuspids and molars continuing as an arc through.

Curve of Wilson

This is a curve that contacts the buccal and lingual cusp tips of the mandibular buccal teeth. It results from inward inclination of the lower posterior teeth.

Curve of Monson

The curve of monson is obtained by extending the curve of spee. It is curve of wilson to all cusps and incisal edges.

CENTRIC RELATION AND CENTRIC OCCLUSION

Centric Relation

Centric relation is the relation of the mandible to the maxilla when the mandibular condyles are in the most superior and retruded position in their glenoid fossa with the articular disk properly interposed.

Centric Occlusion

Centric occlusion is that position of the mandibular condyle when the teeth are in maximum intercuspation.

THE TEMPOROMANDIBULAR JOINTS

The temporomandibular joint is the articulation between the squamous part of the temporal bone and the head of the mandibular condyle.

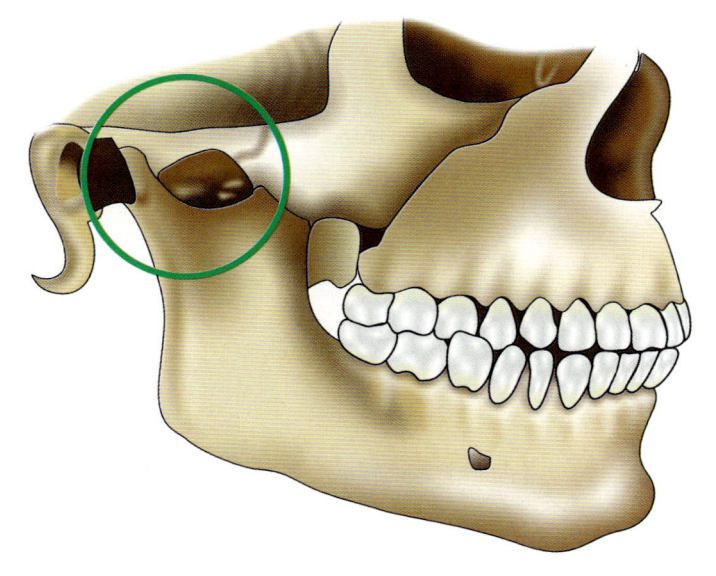

Fig. 18.41

Types of Joint

i. Multiaxial
ii. Bicondylar
iii. Synovial
iv. Ginglimoid.

Bones Involved in the TMJ

Temporal Bone

The glenoid fossa on the mandibular fossa found on the under surface of the squamous part of the temporal bone forms one of the components of the temporomandibular joint.

The Mandibular Condyle

The condyle is the articulating surface of the mandible that consists of the articulating head and a constricted portion below it called the neck of the condyle.

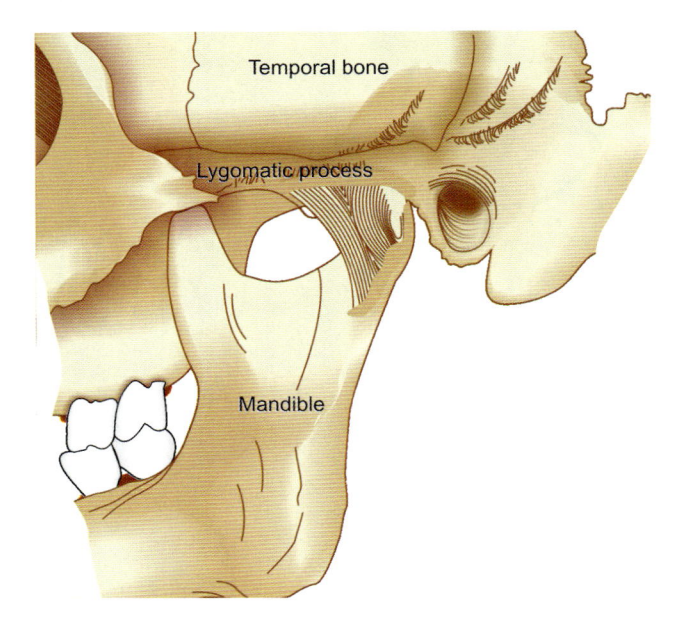

Fig. 18.42

Fibrous Capsule

The temporomandibular joint is enclosed in a thick fibrous capsule.

Articular Disk

The articular disk on meniscus is an oval shaped fibrous plate found between the two articulating bary surfaces, i.e. the condyle and the mandibular fossa. The articular disk divides the joint space into a superior and inferior synovial cavity.

Introduction of Dentition 241

Intra-articular disk

Ligament
Bone

Temporomandibular joint (TMJ)

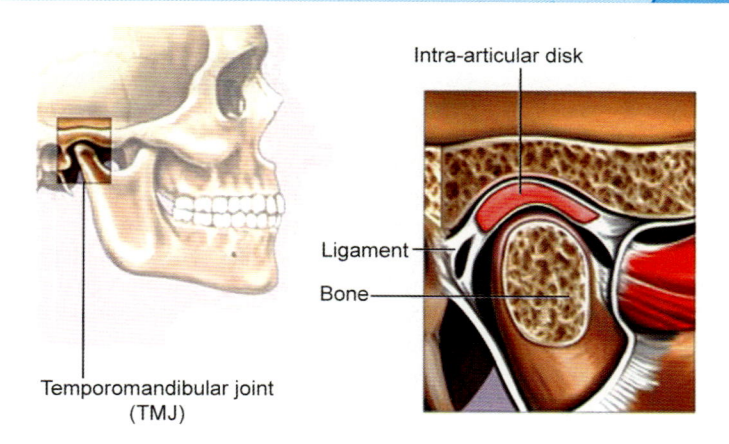

Fig. 18.43

Temporalis muscle

Masseter muscle

Digastric muscle

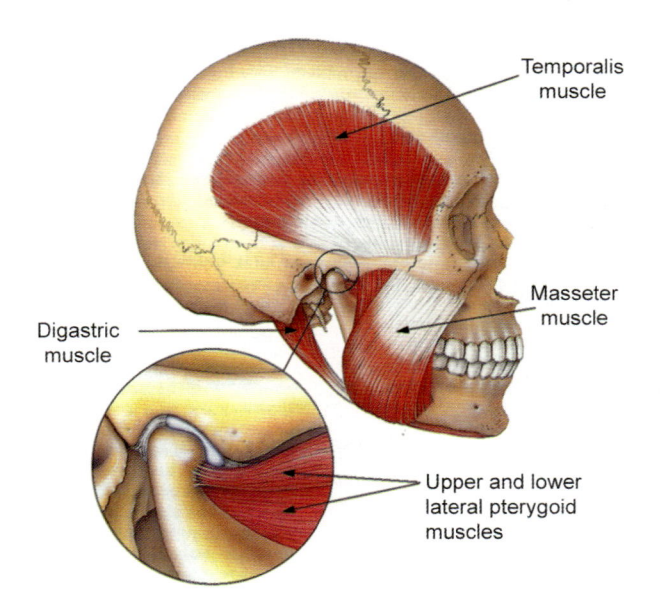

Upper and lower lateral pterygoid muscles

Fig. 18.44

242 Dental Anatomy

Table 18.5: Muscles, action during various jaw movements

Sl. No.	Action	Muscle involved
1.	Depression	• Lateral pterygoid • Digastric, geniohyoid and mylohyoid for opening wide against resistance
2.	Elevation	• Temporalis, masseter and medial pterygoid
3.	Protrusion	• Lateral pterygoid, medial pterygoid
4.	Retrussion	• Posterior fibers of temporalis, assisted by masseter, digastric and geniohyoid
5.	Side to side	• Medial and lateral pterygoid of each side acting alternatively

Protrusion
• Lateral pterygoid assisted by medial pterygoid

Retraction
• Posterior fibers of temporalis, deep part of masseter, and geniohyoid and digastric

Elevation
• Temporalis, masseter, medial pterygoid

Depression
• Gravity
• Digastric, geniohyoid, and mylohyoid muscles

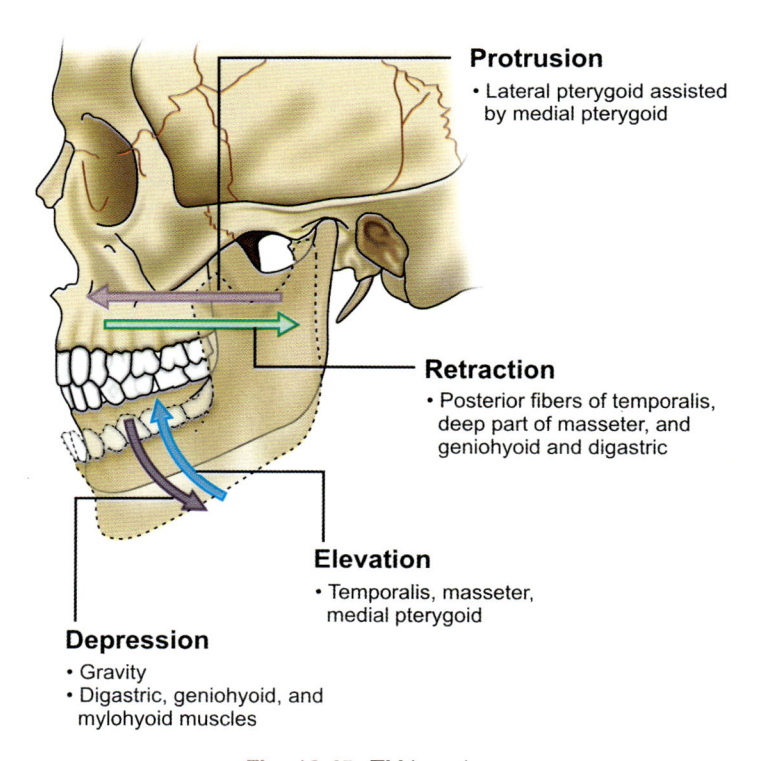

Fig. 18.45: TMJ motions

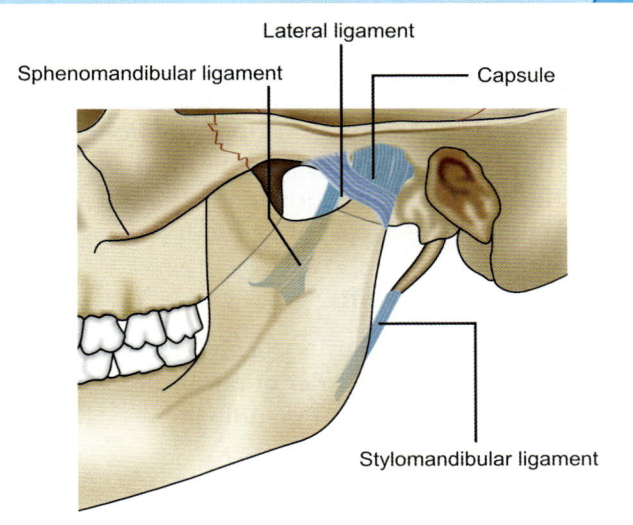

Fig. 18.46: Ligaments intercalated with the TMJ

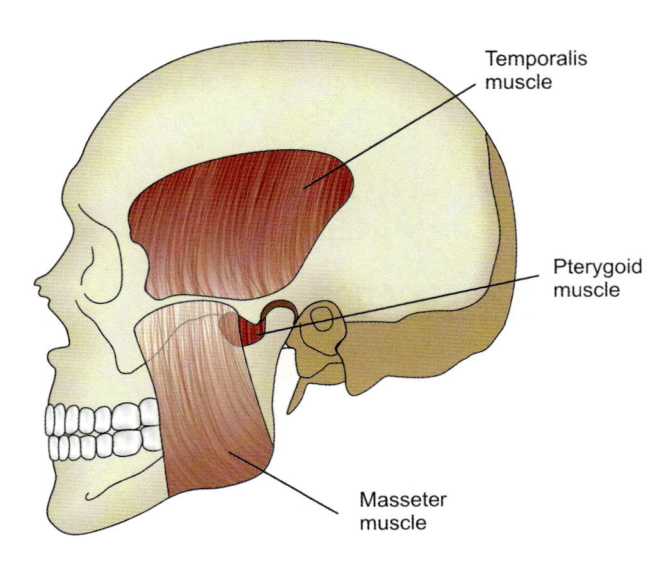

Fig. 18.47: Muscles of mastication

LIGAMENTS INTERCALATED WITH THE TMJ

Sphenomandibular Ligament

It is an accessory ligament as it does not contribute to the stability of the TMJ. It functions to limit the over movement of the mandible. Attached superiorly to the spine of sphenoid and inferiorly to the medial aspect of vamus.

Stylomandibular Ligament

Attached above the lateral surface of styloid process and below to the angle and posterior border of ramus of mandible. It also helps to limit the movement of mandible.

Blood Supply

Anterior	-	Temporal artery
		Masseteric artery
Posteromedial	-	Auricular artery
		Tympanic artery
		Middle meningeal artery
Posterior and Lateral	-	Superficial temporal artery
		Tranverse facial artery

Nerve Supply

Anterior	-	Masseteric nerve
Posterior	-	Auriculotemporal nerve

MUSCLES OF MASTICATION

The muscles of mastications are:
1. Masseter
2. Temporalis
3. Medial pterygoid
4. Lateral pterygoid

It helps during mastication of food and speech. They are derived from first branchial arch. The nerve supply is by mandibular branch of trigeminal nerve.

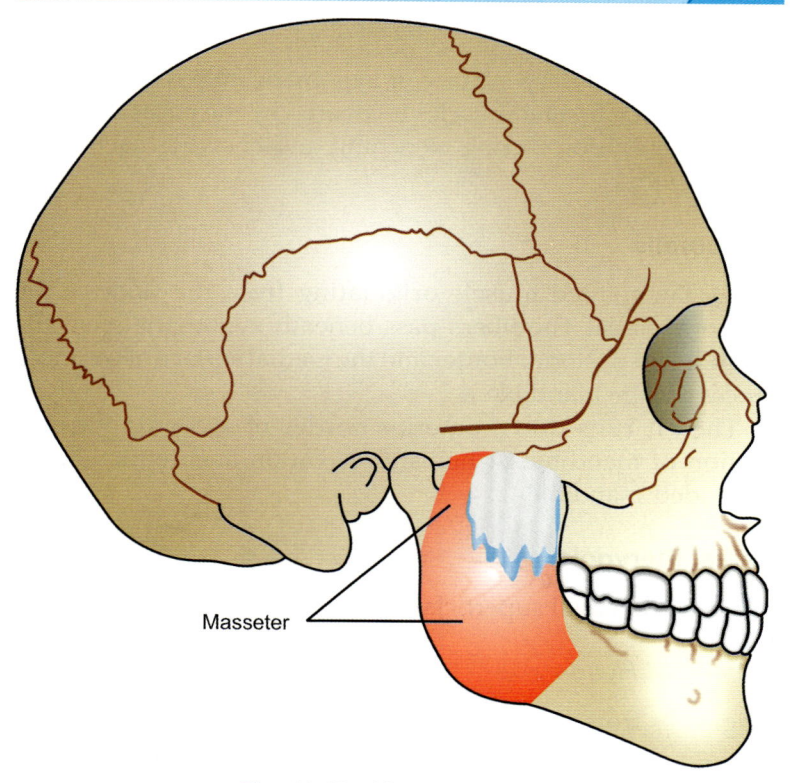

Fig. 18.48: Masseter muscle

Masseter

It lies over the ramus of the mandible.

Superficial Layer

Arises anterior 2/3rd of the lower border of the zygomatic arch and zygomatic process of the maxilla.

Middle Layer

Anterior 2/3rd of the deep surface and posterior 1/3rd of lower border of zygomatic arch.

Deep Layer

Originates from deep surface of zygomatic arch.

A part of masseter muscles is covered by the parotid land. It helps in elevation during clenching and chewing. Action by protrussion.

Temporalis

It is a fan shaped muscle originating from the floor of the temporal fossa. The fibers pass beneath zygomatic arch, the anterior and posterior border and the medial surface of coronoid process of the mandible.

Then it runs down anterior border of ascending ramus portion of mandible. It helps in elevation and retractions of protruded mandible.

Medial Pterygoid

It consists of small superficial head and a large deep head.

Superficial Head

Originates from maxillary tuberosity and palatine bone.

Deep Head

Originates from medial surface of lateral pterygoid plate of the splenoid bone.

The fibers are attached to the angle of mandible. It helps in elevation and protrussion.

Lateral Pterygoid

It also consists of superior head and inferior head.

Superior Head

It is small and originates from infratemporal surface and crest of greater wing of the sphenoid bone.

Introduction of Dentition 247

Inferior Head

Originates from lateral surface of the lateral pterygoid plate.

The two heads pass backward and outward towards the temporomandibular joint and insert into pterygoid fovea of the mandibular condyle, articular disk and capsule. It helps in jaw opening and protrussion.

BLOOD AND NERVE SUPPLY OF THE DENTITION

Blood Supply

The arterial supply of jaw and dentitions are derived from terminal branches of large blood vessels.

The common carotid artery divides into external carotid artery and internal carotid artery. The external carotid artery gives rise to facial artery, lingual artery and the maxillary artery.

The arterial supply of the jaws and dentition is derived from maxillary artery. The facial artery supplies the skin and muscles of the facial region.

The lingual artery supplies the tongue and the floor of the oral cavity.

The inferior alveolar and the superior alveolar arteries are the branches of maxillary artery that supplies the dentitions and the jaws.

Inferior alveolar artery supplies to the molar region of mandible. The inferior alveolar nerve branch out as mental nerve and supplies premolar and anterior tooth of the mandible.

The posterior superior alveolar artery supply the maxillary posterior teeth.

The infraorbital artery branches out to the middle superior alveolar artery and the anterior superior alveolar artery which supplies to the maxillary premolar and incisor teeth and the supporting tissues.

The greater palatine and lesser palatine arteries and the branches of maxillary artery which supplies to the palatal mucosa, lingual gingiva, and soft palate.

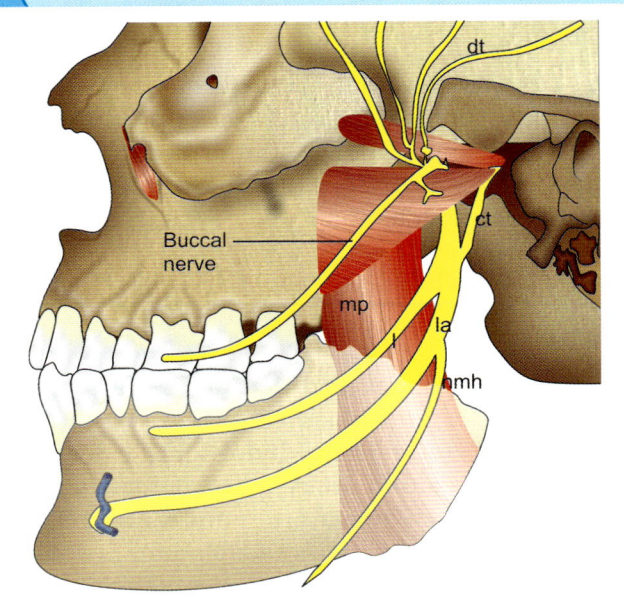

Fig. 18.49

Venous Drainage of Teeth

Most of the veins follow the same pathways as the arteries and may therefore have similar names.

The superior alveolar artery either drain anteriorly to join the facial vein or posteriorly to the pterygoid venous plexus. The facial vein joins the anterior retromandibular vein to form the common facial vein which again joins the internal jugular vein.

Lymphatic Drainage

The lymphatic system comprises of tiny channels connected together by nodular structures called lymph nodes. The system functions by returning the fluids to the blood stream from the various tissues of the body.

The lymph vessels draining the pulp and periodontal ligament have a common outlet. The lymph vessels of all teeth,

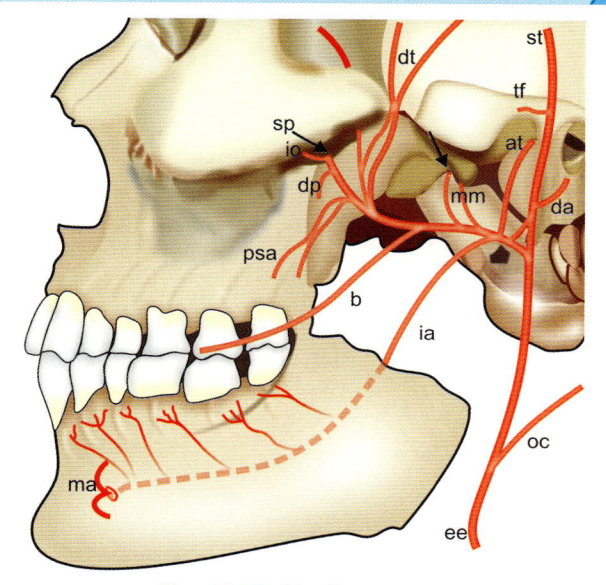

Fig. 18.50: Maxillary artery

except the lower incisors pass into the submandibular lymph nodes of the same side. The lower incisors drain into the submental lymph nodes.

The palatal gingiva drain into the jugulodigastric lymph nodes.

Nerve Supply to the Dentition

The sensory innervation of the jaws, teeth, the mucous membrane lining the vestibule and oral cavity proper is from the maxillary and mandibular divisions of Trigeminal nerve.

The posterior superior alveolar nerve, middle superior and anterior superior alveolar nerves supplies the innervation to the total maxillary teeth.

The inferior alveolar nerve, mental nerve and incisive branches supplies innervation to the total mandibular teeth and the supporting structures. In addition buccal and lingual nerves contribute to some extent.

Section 4

Histochemistry

Histochemistry of Oral Tissue

Chapter 19

CHEMICAL COMPONENTS OF ORAL TISSUE

Oral tissues are composed of:
- Epithelial lining (Epithelium)
- Connective tissues
- Associated muscle fibers.

Epithelium

- Epithelial cells show presence of glycogen in superficial layers with protein and carbohydrates in the cytoplasm.
- Basal lamina as composed of type IV collagen fibroids, laminin, fibronectin and proteoglycans.
- Salivary gland contains mucins or mucoids, which contains proteoglycans and glycoproteins. Histochemical detection of mucins is generally based on their glycosaminoglycan content, which affects the staining reaction.
- The acidic nature is due to presence of glucuronic acid, sulfate or sialic acids.

Connective Tissues

- This is of mesenchymal origin and consists of various types of cells and fibers, embedded in amorphous semigel and colloidal ground substance.

Histochemistry

- The ground substance is made of proteoglycans and glycoproteins secreted by cells like fibroblasts and mast cells.
- Proteoglycans can be sulfated like chondroitin sulfates, keratin sulfates and heparin sulfates or can be nonsulfated like hyaluronic acid.
- Glycoproteins are protein molecules with lesser number of carbohydrate molecules than in proteoglycans. Glycoproteins are named as fibronectin, laminin, chondronectin and astorectin.
- Glycoproteins help in cell attachment to the extracellular matrix and thus are responsible for the maintenance of normal cell morphology and also controlled cell function.
- Change in concentration is seen in conditions like inflammation, early stages of wound healing and cancer.
- Histochemistry is the main tool of investigating enzymatic reactions in the cells. Most commonly used are, acid and alkaline phosphatases, oxidases, dehydrogenases, esterases and other enzymes involved in the metabolic activities of the cells.

Histochemical Analysis of Oral Soft Tissue

- Various chemical components of cells can be visualized by staining reactions or formation of insoluble dye or precipitate at the reaction life.

Carbohydrates

- Most common staining method used for the study of glycogen, proteoglycans and glycoproteins is PAS (periodic acid-Schiff) reaction.
- When periodic acid is treated with leucofuchsin (Schiff's reagent), it oxidizes the glycol groups to aldehyde and produce reddish purple dye product.
- PAS is used to study epithelial mucopolysaccharides, basement membrane and mucus of salivary glands.
- Basement membrane can also be studied by silver methenamine and oxidation of aldehyde group.

Histochemistry of Oral Tissue

- Salivary mucins can be stained by mucicarmine.
- Metachromatic stain toluidine blue is used for demonstration of proteoglycans and metachromatic reactive bromine purple to red is produced depending upon the degree of polymerization of the dye molecules.
- Metachromatic reaction is also used for demonstration of mast cells, which are rich in heparin and for intercellular ground substance of young bone and cartilage.

Mucins

- Salivary mucins are composed of high molecular weight carbohydrate protein complexes.
- **Mucins are of two types:**
  - Falco mucin—rich and - fucose
  - Siab mucin—rich in sialic acid.
- Mucicarmine and mucihematin used for nonspecific staining of mucin (neutral mucins) are identified by PAS technique.
- Acid mucins are localized by blue, toluidine blue, colloidal iron and aldehyde fuchsin method.
- Alcian blue stain used for the mucins.

Proteins

- These groups are demonstrated histochemically by ferric-ferricyanide method.
- Red colored reaction product is formed on reaction with dinitrofluorobenzene (DNFB) and ninhydrin in Schiff reagent.

Lipids

- Frozen sections are used for study of lipids and staining with sudan black or oil red is employed.

Enzymes

- It carried out on Frozen sections. Reaction is done at 37°C, the temperature at which enzymes are active *in vivo*.

- The reaction is made visible with the help of cobalt or lead compounds and end product is insoluble black.

Alkaline phosphatase
- Present in capillary endothelium of lamina proper basement membranes associated with salivary gland acin show high alkaline phosphatase activity.

Acid phosphatase
- Related to the degree of keratinization. It is very high in the zone of keratinization and is low in non-keratinized areas.

Esterase
- Some esterase activity is present in superficial layers. High activity is present on salivary gland ducts and also in serous demilunes of the sublingual gland.
- Also present in taste buds and mast cells of oral tissues.

Cytochrome oxidase
- Histochemical techniques show low levels of cytochrome oxidase activity in human gingiva.
- Localized in basal layers of the free and attached gingiva, curricular epithelium and epithelial attachment.
- Increase in cytochrome activity is observed in chronic gingivitis. It is also seen in salivary duct system.
- Differentiation of connective tissues components like collagen and muscle is carried out on the basis of pore size and permeability of fixed tissues and molecular size of the anionic dyes.
- Collagen has bigger pore compared to muscle so reacts with bigger molecular size in the trichrome stains like von Gieson and masson's trichrome.
- In von Gieson stain, collagen stains red and muscle takes yellow.
- In Masson's trichrome stain, collagen stains green or blue depending on the dye and muscle stains red.
- Reticular and elastic fibers have strong affinity for liver, so demonstrated by liver impregnation techniques.

Histochemical Analysis of Oral Hard Tissues

Carbohydrates

- Most common technique in the study of ground substance of bone and teeth is PAS stain to demonstrate carbohydrates.
- This can demonstrate the developing and resorting bone and dentin by stronger PAS reactivity than mature tissues.
- Poorly calcified dentin mature in interlobular dentin, dentinogenous imorfecta and in odontomas show distinct PAS reaction.
- Enamel is nonreactive with PAS but enamel lamellae stain intensely.

Proteins

- Dentin proteins undergoing decay and in developmental stages stain intensely with histochemical reaction.
- Two important methods are dinitrofluorobenzene (DNFB) and ninhydrin Schiff methods.
- DNFB forms pale yellow complex. Azo dye is formed to give up deep red color.
- In the ninhydrin Schiff method, Schiff reagent reacts and form a red colored product.

Lipids

- Important methods are DNFB and ninhydrin schiff method.
- Mature dentin shows low lipid content but enamel rod sheaths and odontoblastic processes are strongly sudanophilic due to high phospholipid content.
- Sudnophilia depends on the solubility of sudan dyes with lipids. In developing tooth, this dye is seen in zone of mineralization and predentin and in the basal zone of the ameloblasts which indicates the role of phospholipids in the process of mineralization of dentin and enamel matrix.

Enzymes

Alkaline phosphates
- Activity is seen in endosteum, periosteum, osteocytes, stratum intermedium, odontoblasts, Korff's fibers and the ground substance of developing molars and incisors.
- It is associated with process of mineralization, osteogenesis and dentinogenesis. It gives an intense staining in case of osteoblasts and odontoblasts.

Acid phosphatase
- Localized in osteoclasts and odontoclast lying in the resorting surface of bone and dentin. Mainly localized in membrane bound organelles, the lysosomes.

Esterase
- By the use of specific naphthol esters like naphthol acetate, intense staining reaction is seen in calcifying matrix of bone and dentin.
- Activity of esterase can be appreciated in the cells and microorganisms associated with formation of calculus deposits on teeth.

Cytochrome oxidase
- Enables cells to utilize molecular oxygen. It shows the oxygen requirement and their metabolic and physiologic activity.
- Osteoblasts and osteoclasts show oxidase activity. It can also be seen in stratum intermedium of molars and incisors.
- Other enzymes detected are succinate dehydrogenase and α-ketoglutaric dehydrogenase.

IMMUNOHISTOCHEMISTRY

Introduction
- Chemicals in our body have the ability to stain in a different manner.
- Information about normal and pathologic conditions of the tissues can be obtained by histochemical and other advanced techniques.

Histochemistry of Oral Tissue — 259

Immunofluorescence is a method to detect the biomolecules, cytoplasmic fibers, antigens, nuclei and other structures.
- Monoclonal antibodies developed against is elucidated with the help of fluorescence probes like fluorescein isothiocyanate (FITC).
- The technique is simple and extremely sensitive; special microscope is required for visualization. Now a days immunoperoxidase technique is used where marker for elucidating the reaction is enzyme hopse-padish peroxidase.
- Brown insoluble precipitate is formed at the life of reaction which can be visualized with light microscope.
- Main advantage of this method is versatility. Immunofluorescence can be used on frozen tissues, immunoperoxidase can be used on paraffin embedded tissues also.
- Immunofluorescence have to be examined immediately and cannot be presented. Immunoperoxidase sections can be mounted and presented for long time sections can also be studied on electron microscope.

OTHER ADVANCED TECHNIQUES

- Biomolecules play important role in normal tissues development, function and pathologic conditions.
- To detect biomolecules, special techniques are needed biochemical investigations are useful in determining normal and abnormal concentration of biomolecules, enzymes, etc.
- Histochemical techniques are of immense importance in providing in light into the biochemical changes taking place inside the cell and their relationship with the structural components.
- Molecular biology is playing increasingly important role and techniques of immunohistochemistry, in which hybridization, immunofluorescence are being used.

CLINICAL CONSIDERATION

- Very important in the diagnosis of oral lesions.
- It is mostly applied on salivary gland tumors arriving from the nonglandular epithelium mucopolysaccharides demonstrated in the fungi, like candidiasis, histoplasmosis, actinomycolis, blastomycosis and coccidiomycosis.
- Can also be used for tumors arising from tat cells like lipoma and liposarcoma.

Microtechnique

Chapter 20

MICROTECHNIQUE

[Preparation of specimens for Histologic study]

The ultimate test of all dental education is to see how well it prepares the practitioner to serve the patient.

Undoubtedly good treatment is doing good service to patient.

What is the Treatment?

To manage the patient with care, to change the abnormal conditions to the normal conditions.

When will it be a Success?

The practitioner should have a thorough knowledge of the normal and abnormal conditions, that means the histological and pathological conditions of the body.

So the study of the histological and pathological conditions of the hard and soft tissues is very important.

How will we Study these Conditions?

"Under Microscope" we study the histological and pathological conditions of the body.

Tissues for light microscopic study must be sufficiently thin to transmit light, and its components must have sufficient contrast for the parts to be distinguishable from each other.

Histochemistry

So the preparation of the material (slide) from oral tissues, for study under microscope is necessary.

This process of preparation is called microtechnique.

IMPORTANCE OF MICROTECHNIQUE

Microtechnique is the basic way to study and diagnose the diseased conditions in cells (Cytology), (Cellular Pathology) and tissues (Histopathology).

It helps to plan the line of treatment.

Microtechnique can play a vital role in providing medico-legal clues in cases of suspected and mysterious circumstances.

METHODS OF MICROTECHNIQUE

There are four methods of microtechnique:
  I. Preparation of sections of paraffin embedded specimens (soft tissues).
  II. Preparation of sections of parlodion embedded specimens (hard tissues).
  III. Preparation of ground sections of teeth and bone.
  IV. Preparation of frozen sections.

Steps in Preparation of Sections of:

  I. Paraffin embedded specimens (soft tissues).
  II. Parlodion embedded specimens (hard tissues).
  1. Obtaining the specimen.
  2. Fixation.
  3. Decalcification.
  4. Dehydration and clearing.
  5. Infiltration and Impregnation.
  6. Embedding.
  7. Sectioning.
  8. Mounting.
  9. Staining.

Obtaining the Specimen

Specimens taken from patients must be removed carefully without crushing.

If it is hard tissue, the unwanted soft tissue is removed and better to cut into several pieces before placing it in the fixative because a smaller specimen allows quicker penetration of the fixing solutions to its center.

Fixation

Immediately after removal of the specimen it must be placed in fixing solution.

The purposes of fixation are to preserve as nearly as possible the natural state of the tissue cells.

The most widely used fixative is 10% formalin [commercial formalin (full strength) – 10 ml and distilled water – 90 ml].

Other than formalin, the Zenker's fluid, Bouins fluid, Carnoy's fluid and Helly's fluid are available for special purposes.

Period: The fixation period varies from several hours to several days, depending on the size and density of the specimens, and on the types of fixing solution used.

After fixation, the specimen is washed overnight in running water.

Decalcification

When preparing sections of calcified tissues like bone and teeth, decalcification is necessary in order to facilitate cutting.

One way of decalcification is to suspend the specimen in about 400 ml of 5% nitric acid.

The acid is changed daily for 8 to 10 days.

Other methods of decalcification:
  i. Ion exchange method.
  ii. Chelation method, and
  iii. Electrical ionization method.

How to test the specimen for decalcification?

i. One way to test for complete decalcification is to pierce the hard tissue with a needle, when the needle enters the bone and tooth easily the tissue is probably ready for further treatment.

ii. Another way to test for complete decalcification is to determine by a precipitation test. Ammonium hydroxide and ammonium oxalate are used for this test.

When decalcification is complete the specimen must be washed in running water for at least 24 hours.

Dehydration

The process of removal of water from the specimen is called dehydration. It is necessary that the specimen be completely infiltrated with the paraffin or parlodion.

Dehydration is accomplished by the placement of the specimen successively in increasing percentages of alcohol (40%, 60%, 80%, 95%, and absolute alcohol).

The specimen should remain in each of the alcohol including 95% for 24 to 48 hours and it should be placed in several changes of absolute alcohol over a period of 48 to 72 hours.

Clearing

The process of dealcoholization (removal of alcohol) is known as clearing.

The hard tissue specimen from the absolute alcohol is transferred to ether alcohol and xylene respectively.

Infiltration and Impregnation

The soft tissue specimen removed from xylene is ready to be infiltrated with paraffin.

This soft tissue is placed in a dish of melted embedding paraffin, and the dish is put into a constant temperature oven regulated to about 60°C.

The specimen is changed to two or three successive dishes of paraffin, so that all of the xylene in the tissue is replaced by paraffin.

The hard tissue specimen from ether alcohol is transferred to 2% parlodion, covered tightly to prevent evaporation and allowed to stand for a period of 2 weeks to a month.

From 2% parlodion, the specimen is transferred to increasing percentages of parlodion (4%, 6%, 10%, and 12%).

The infiltration time of specimen depends upon the size and density of the specimen.

Embedding

The hard and soft tissue specimens are completely infiltrated and they are embedded in the center of a block of paraffin and parlodion respectively with the help of Leuckart embedding boxes.

Sectioning

The microtome is used for sectioning the specimen.
Commonly used microtomes are:
  i. Rotary microtome.
  ii. Cambridge rocking microtome.
  iii. Cryostat.
  iv. Freezing microtome.

The specimen block is attached to the metal object holder of microtome.

The microtome is adjusted to cut sections to the desired thickness (usually 4 to 10 μm) and the perfectly sharpened microtome knife is clamped into place for sectioning.

This sharpened microtome knife cut the tissue to desired thickness on the rotation of the microtome.

Mounting-I

The soft tissue sections are mounted on prepared microscope slides with the help of Meyer's albumin adhesive.

Meyer's albumin is a combination of egg albumin and glycerin.

The hard tissue sections are not mounted on slides until after staining, dehydration and clearing are completed.

Instead of Meyer's albumin, xylene is used as the adhesive in case of the hard tissues mounting.

Staining

Staining of the section enables one to study the physical characteristics and relationship of tissues and of their constituent cells.

The natural dyes, synthetic dyes used for routine, microscopic study is hematoxylin and eosin, commmonly known as H and E.

Other methods of staining
1. Gomori's method
2. Periodic acid Schiff (PAS)
3. The Faulgen method
4. Pyronin and malachite green method.
5. Weigert-von Gieson stain.
6. Masson's trichrome stain.
7. Silver impregnation method.

Mounting II

The stained sections are covered with a mounting medium [(i) Canada Balsam (or) (ii) DPX] and a cover glass is affixed when the mounting medium has hardened. The slides are ready for examination.

Preparation of Frozen Sections

Fixed soft tissues or fresh unfixed soft tissues may be cut into sections 10 to 15 μm thick by freezing the block of tissue with either liquid or solid carbon dioxide and cutting on a freezing microtome.

Uses of Frozen Sections

Frozen sections can be quickly prepared and are useful if the immediate examination of a specimen is required.

Preparation of Ground Sections of Teeth or Bone

Undecalcified teeth or bone may be studied by making ground sections of the specimens.

After extraction, the extracted teeth should be preserved in 10% formalin.

With the help of the coarse and fine abrasive lathe wheel which is attached to the laboratory lathe, make thin sections.

The stained/unstained ground sections are useful in study of teeth and bones.

Index

A

Age changes in
  alveolus 152
  cementum 151
  dentin 149
    vital tissue 149
  dento-gingival function 152
  enamel 148
  mandible 147
    in adults 147
    in infants and children 147
    in old age 147
  oral mucosa 152
  periodontal ligament 151
  pulp 149
  salivary glands 152
  TM joint and maxillary sinus 152
Alveolar process 86
  alveolar bone proper 86
  supporting bone 86

B

Bilaminar germ disk 6
Blood and nerve supply of dentition 247
  blood supply 247
  lymphatic drainage 248
  nerve supply to dentition 249
  venous drainage of teeth 248
Bone cells 87
  osteoblasts 87
  osteoclasts 88
  osteocytes 88
Bone formation 83
  composition of bone 84
  structure of bone 85
  types 83
    endochondral bone formation 83
    intramembranous bone formation 84
Bony remodelling theory 137
Branchial arches and primitive mouth 9
Buccopharyngeal membrane 7, 9

C

Calcium 177
  absorption 178
  calcium excretion 180
  calcium regulation 180
  functions 180
  types 178
Cementum 70
  cementoblasts 71
  cementodentinal junction 73
  cementoenamel junction 73
  cementogenesis 71
  cementoid 72
  clinical considerations 75
  function 74
  hypercementosis 74
  physical characteristics 70
  structure 72
Chemical components of oral tissue 253
  connective tissues 253
  epithelium 253
  histochemical analysis of oral hard tissues 257
  histochemical analysis of oral soft tissue 254

Textbook of Human Oral Embryology, Anatomy...

Chronology of mandibular first
    molar 233
    buccal aspect 233
    distal aspect 234
    lingual aspect 233
    mesial aspect 234
    occlusal aspect 235
Compound exocytosis 110
    applied aspect 113
    identification of mucous
        glands 113
    identification point of serous
        cell 110
    mucous cells 111
Cortical plate 86
Cranial nerves 160
Cribriform plate 87
Crown-rump length 4

D

Deciduous tooth germs 133
Dental lamina 17
    fate of dental lamina 18
Dental occlusion 236
Dental papilla 19, 21, 23
Dental sac 19, 21, 23
Dentin 42
    age changes in dentin 52
        dead tracts 52
        reparative dentin 53
        sclerotic dentin 53
    development 43
        formation of matrix 43
        mineralization 44
    innervation of dentin 53
        direct nerve stimulation
            theory 53
        hydrodynamic theory 54
        odontoblast receptor
            theory 54
    physical properties 42
        composition 43
    structural lines 51

contour lines of own 52
incremental lines of von
    Ebner 51
mineralizing lines 51
neonatal line 51
structures of dentin 44
    circumpulpal dentin 49
    dentinal tubules 44
    dentinoenamel junction 46
    granular layer of tomes 50
    intertubular dentin 46
    intratubular (peritubular
        dentin) 46
    mantle dentin 47
    predentin 50
    primary dentin 48
    secondary dentin 49
Derivatives of germ layers and
    neural crest 7
Development of face 10
Development of mandible 14
Development of maxilla 15
Development of secondary palate
    11
Development of temporomandi-
    bular joint 16
Development of skull 13
Development of tongue 12

E

Effects of growth hormone 153
Embryoblast 4
Enamel 28
    chemical properties 29
    physical properties 28
        color 28
        density 29
        hardness 28
        permeability 28
        solubility 29
        tensile strength and
            compressibility 29
        thickness 29

Index

structural features 31
   enamel lamellae 33
   enamel spindles 35
   enamel tufts 34
   gnarled enamel 33
   Hunter-Schreger bands 32
   incremental lines of Retzius 31
structure 30
surface structures 35
   enamel cuticle 36
   perikymata 35
Enamel organ 19
Exocytosis 110

F

Facial nerve 168
   course 170
   extracranial course 171
   intracranial branches 171
Fate of grooves and pouches 9
First maxillary molars 228
   buccal aspect 229
   distal aspect 230
   lingual aspect 229
   mesial aspect 230
   occlusal aspect 230
Folding of embryo 7
Formation of neural tube 4
   functions 5
Formation of three-layered embryo 6
Functions of salivary ducts 117
   connective tissue elements 117

G

Gamete cells 3
Ganglion 156
Gingiva 95
   microscopic features 95
      junctional epithelium 96

      outer oral epithelium 96
      sulcular epithelium 96
Gingival sulcus 97
Glossopharyngeal nerve 171
   extracranial course 173
   intracranial course 172
Golgi complex 61

H

Haploid cells 3
Hard palate 93
Hertwig's epithelial root sheath 24
Histology of 134
   eruptive phase 134
   posteruptive phase 135
   pre-eruptive phase 134
Hormones on oral structures 153
   thyroid hormone 153
Hydrostatic pressure theory 137
Hypoglossal nerve 174
   branches 176
   course 174
   origin 174

I

Immunohistochemistry 258
Influence of parathyroid hormone 154
Inner enamel epithelium 22

K

Korff's fibers 43

L

Lamina propria 92
Life cycle of ameloblast 36
   desmolytic stage 41
   formative stage 39
   maturative stage 40
   morphogenic stage 37

organizing stage 37
protective stage 41
Ligaments intercalated with TMJ 244
Line angles and point angles 189
Lines of von Ebner 51
Lymphoid cells 63

M

Malassez 25
Mandibular canine 217
 distal aspect 218
 incisal aspect 218
 labial aspect 218
 lingual aspect 218
 mesial aspect 218
Mandibular central incisor 211
 distal aspect 213
 incisal aspect 213
 labial aspect 211
 lingual aspect 212
 mesial aspect 213
Mandibular first molar 232
Mandibular first premolar 222
 buccal aspect 223
 distal aspect 225
 lingual aspect 224
 mesial aspect 224
 occlusal aspect 225
Mandibular lateral incisor 214
 incisal aspect 215
 labial and lingual aspect 214
 mesial and distal aspect 214
Mandibular nerve 166
 branches 167
 course 166
 origin 166
 relations 167
Mandibular primary central incisors 196
 labial aspect 196
 lingual aspect 197
 mesial and distal aspects 197

Mandibular primary first molar 200
 buccal aspect 201
 distal aspect 202
 lingual aspect 201
 mesial aspect 202
 occlusal aspect 201
 occlusal aspect 202
Mandibular second premolar 226
 buccal aspect 226
 distal aspect 227
 lingual aspect 226
 mesial aspect 227
 occlusal aspect 227
Mandibular third molar 236
Masticatory mucosa 93
Maxillary and mandibular canine 215
 distal aspect 217
 incisal aspect 217
 labial aspect 216
 lingual aspect 216
 mesial aspect 216
Maxillary central incisor 208
 distal aspect 210
 incisal aspect 210
 labial aspect 208
 lingual aspect 209
 mesial aspect 209
Maxillary molars 227
Maxillary nerve 164
 branches 164
 course 164
 relations 164
Maxillary primary canine 197
 labial aspect 198
 lingual aspect 198
 mesial and distal aspect 198
Maxillary primary central incisor 195
 labial aspect 195
 lingual aspect 195
 mesial and distal aspects 195
Maxillary second premolar 220

buccal aspect 220
distal aspect 221
lingual aspect 221
mesial aspect 221
occlusal aspect 221
Maxillary sinus 120
  clinical considerations 124
    developmental anomalies 124
      larger sinuses 124
      oroantral fistula 124
  functions 123
Maxillary third molar 232
Maximally primary first molar 198
  buccal aspect 199
  distal aspect 199
  lingual aspect 199
  mesial aspect 199
  occlusal aspect 200
Meckel's cartilage 14
Meckel's cave 156
Mesial drift 136
Microtechnique 261
  importance 262
  methods 262
Mitosis 3
Movement of teeth 132
  eruptive tooth movement 132
  posteruptive movement 132
  pre-eruptive movement 132
Muscles of mastication 244
  lateral pterygoid 246
  masseter 245
  medial pterygoid 246
  temporalis 246

N

Neural crest cells 5
Neural groove 5

O

Odontogenic epithelium 11
Olfactory placode 10

Ophthalmic nerve 163
Oral cavity 90
  classification 90
    lining mucosa 91
    masticatory mucosa 91
    specialized mucosa 91
  physiology 90
Outer enamel epithelium 23

P

Papillae 100
  filiform papillae 100
  foliate papillae 102
  fungiform papillae 101
  vallate (circumvallate) papillae 102
Parasympathetic ganglia 157
  ciliary ganglion 158
    branches 159
    roots 158
  otic ganglion 159
    geniculate ganglion 159
    situation 159
  pterygopalatine ganglion 158
    branches 158
    motor branches 158
  submandibular ganglion 157
    branch 157
    roots 157
    situation 157
Perifollicular mesenchyme 77
Periodontal ligament 76
  development 77
  functions 78
    formative 78
    nutritive 79
    resorptive 78
    sensory 79
    supportive 78
  other structures 82
    blood vessels 82
    nerves 82
  structure 79
    cells of periodontal

ligament 79
   fibers of periodontal ligament 80
Periodontal ligament traction theory 138
Permanent mandibular incisors 211
Permanent mandibular premolars 222
Permanent maxillary premolar 218
   buccal aspect 219
   lingual aspect 219
   mesial aspect 220
Plexus of Raschkow 54
Premature eruption 138
Primary dentition 193
Pulp 56
   anatomy 56
   blood vessels of pulp 63
   clinical considerations 68
   dental papilla 68
   development of pulp 68
   functions of the pulp 66
   mandibular teeth 57
      cuspids 57
      first premolar 57
      lateral incisor 57
      second premolar 58
   maxillary teeth 56
      central incisor 56
      cuspids 57
      first premolar 57
      lateral incisor 56
      second premolar 57
   nerve supply of pulp 65
   pericytes 64
      functions 64
   pulp organ 58
      coronal pulp 58
      radicular pulp 58
   regressive changes of pulp 66
      classification 66
   structural features 59
      defense cells 63
      fibroblast 62
      functions 63
      intercellular substances 62
      odontoblasts 60
      undifferentiated mesenchymal cells 62

S

Saliva composition and function 118
   clinical considerations 118
   common disease seen 119
Salivary glands 105
   anatomy 105
   development of salivary glands 107
   histology and structure 108
   major salivary glands 105
   minor salivary glands 107
Shedding of deciduous teeth 140
   clinical implications 142
   deciduous teeth remnants 142
      submerged deciduous teeth 143
   events 142
   location 142
   mechanisms 142
   odontoclasts 141
   origin 141
Somatic cell 3
Spongiosa 87
Stellate reticulum 21, 22
Stratum intermedium 22
Structure and function of salivary gland cells 113
   ducts of salivary gland 115
      intercalated duct 115
      striated duct 115
      terminal excretory duct 116
   myoepithelial cells 114
Submucosa 93
Sulcular fluid 97

Index

T

Taste buds 103
Taste determination 104
Teeth 185
   functions 186
   landmarks 187
   tooth surfaces 187
Temporomandibular joint 125, 238
   articular capsule 129
   articular disk 125
      articular space 126
      articular fibrous covering 128
      articular disk 128
   causes 131
   clinical considerations 130
   development of joint 127
   dislocation 131
   features 130
   histological features 127
      bony structures 127
   innervation and blood supply 130
   treatment 131

Theories of tooth eruption 136
T-lymphocytes 63
Tomes' granular layer 45
Tooth development 18
   developmental stages 18
      bell stage 22
      bud stage 19
      cap stage 19
Tooth numbering systems 191
Trigeminal ganglion 156
Trigeminal nerve 160

V

Ventral surface of tongue 100
Vestibule and alveolar mucosa 99

Z

Zonula occludens 61
Zsigmondy/palmar notation 193
Zygoma 15
Zygote 3

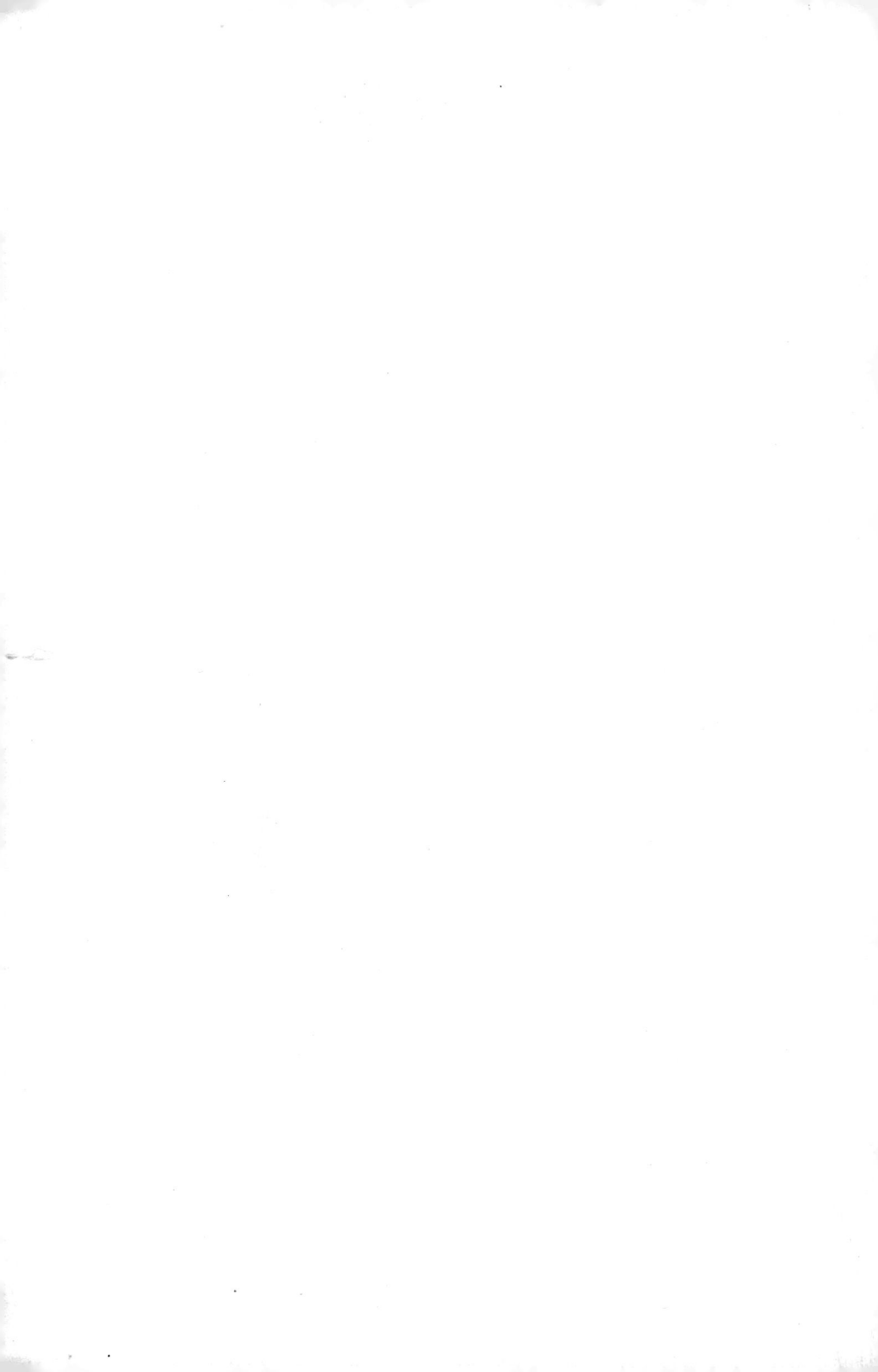